Paediatrics

Paediatrics

N. D. Barnes, MA, MB, B.CHIR, FRCP,
and
N. R. C. Roberton, MA, MB,
B.CHIR, FRCP

Consultant Paediatricians
Addenbrooke's Hospital
Cambridge

1981 Update Books
LONDON

Available in the United Kingdom and Eire from
MTP Press Ltd
Falcon House
Cable Street
Lancaster LA1 1PE
England

Available in the USA and Canada from
Kluwer Boston Inc.
Lincoln Building
160 Old Derby Street
Hingham, Mass. 02043,
USA

Available in the rest of the world from
MTP Press Ltd, England

British Library Cataloguing in Publication Data

Barnes, N. D.
Paediatrics.
1. Pediatrics
I. Title II. Roberton, N. R. C.
618.9'2 RJ45

First Published 1981

Softcover reprint of the hardcover 1st edition 1981

ISBN-13: 978-94-009-7426-5 e-ISBN-13: 978-94-009-7424-1
DOI: 10.1007/978-94-009-7424-1

Contents

Preface

When asked by students of medicine to name a reliable, readable and adequately comprehensive text book of clinical paediatrics we have, in the past, been forced to recommend the least unsatisfactory among the large number of not quite good enough books on the market. Those available always seemed to be too long or too brief, too dogmatic or too discursive, too practical or not practical enough, too selective or too all-embracing. Despairing of this, many of us have attempted writing books of our own only to discover how difficult it is to find the right formula for the general reader seeking a text to reinforce his particular clinical experience. The paragon among books that we would all wish to lay our hands on will probably never be written, but this book, written by my colleagues in Cambridge Dr Nick Barnes and Dr Cliff Roberton, comes very close to the ideal and is certainly my best buy in its category. From it we receive succinct, convincing and helpful accounts of nearly all the conditions affecting children that matter in practice in the sense that ignorance of their existence, importance and significance would materially affect our competence. The writers are obviously extraordinarily well read in the relevant original papers; unlike many learned authors, they have a good nose for the relevant fact and a sure sense of proportion. Their tone of voice, while authoritative, is not provokingly dogmatic and does not challenge accepted truth without justification. One suspects that most readers with experience of paediatric practice will find little of substance to quarrel with in the advice given and in the authors' choice of content, and their style renders what they say unambiguous and often memorable. It is a pleasure for a new colleague to be able to recommend publicly Dr Barnes' and Dr Roberton's book as not only the best we have but, of its kind, as good as we are ever likely to see. It is a fit companion for Dr Chiswick's book, *Neonatal Medicine,* in the same series and for once an addition to the library which will surely appeal to and find a wide readership.

Professor John A. Davis,
Department of Paediatrics,
Cambridge University Medical School.

Foreword

The purpose of this book is to assist in the assessment and management of ill children outside hospital. It is not a short textbook of paediatrics and, freed from the constraints imposed by the need to be comprehensive, we have been able to concentrate on those conditions which seem most important in the context of primary care. Common problems are discussed at some length but no mention is made of rarities seldom encountered in practice. The reader will therefore search in vain for an account of tumours in childhood or inborn errors of metabolism; the general practitioner is unlikely to see a new case of most such conditions in a clinical lifetime and indeed, if he does so, wide experience of normal children and familiarity with the common pattern of disease will generally enable him to detect promptly such unusual problems and to refer them without delay. Investigation and treatment conducted in hospital is considered briefly. We have also omitted consideration of those problems specific to the newborn infant because these were well covered in Dr Malcolm Chiswick's book in this series, *Neonatal Medicine.*

The book is based on a series of articles originally written for *Update* magazine. In each of these we took a single major topic and tried to cover those aspects of most practical importance in the front-line medical care of children. The chapters have all been revised, some added and much new material included.

Our view of the field is seen from the 'sheltered' environment of a hospital paediatric department; we feel that the wide experience of serious disease in childhood so gained offers a vantage point from which the important may be distinguished from the trivial, but we are acutely aware that some might argue that all such views are distorted by distance!

Although we have addressed ourselves primarily to the general practitioner, we have kept the concerns of the medical student in mind, not least because we were inaugurating the clinical paediatric teaching of the Cambridge medical school while writing the book. We hope that the book may also prove useful to paediatric nurses, health visitors and others concerned with the medical care of children. A great deal of factual information is presented in somewhat compressed form but we hope that we have also been able to convey some sense of our own pleasure in working with children, surely the most rewarding of all raw materials available to the medical craftsman.

We would greatly appreciate comments, criticisms and suggestions from readers and will be disappointed only if we fail to provoke any reaction.

Nick Barnes
Cliff Roberton

1. Growth and Growth Problems

In man the journey from conception to physical maturity occupies almost a quarter of the life span. Knowledge of the normal variations of growth and development and the interactions of disease with this orderly process is fundamental to the medicine of childhood. In the unbiased opinion of the authors, it also provides the extra dimension which separates the fascination of paediatrics from the drudgery of adult medicine!

Although the complexity of human growth and its control is overwhelming, the salient facts relevant to the clinical assessment of growth disorders can be summarized simply. In this chapter we will consider some aspects of the biology of human growth and discuss the application of these principles in the clinical assessment, diagnosis and management of growth problems in childhood.

The Biology of Growth

Prenatal Growth

This is the period of growth about which least is known and yet it is the most important, since the development of organ systems and the most rapid increase in cell number occur before birth. Prenatal growth can be subdivided into two phases.

1. Embryonic growth, which occupies the first eight weeks of fetal life and encompasses the chief era of organogenesis.

2. Fetal growth, from eight weeks to full term, during which there is elaboration of the function of organ systems and rapid growth in size of the fetus. The most rapid growth in length occurs at about 20 weeks and in weight at about 34 weeks gestation, so growth is already slowing at the time of birth. The maternal, placental and fetal factors which control prenatal growth are poorly understood but the effects of growth-retarding processes at this stage of development are often irrecoverable. For many children with problems of growth the die was cast long before birth and the aim must be prevention rather than cure.

Postnatal Growth

The familiar linear growth curve, in which height attained is expressed against age, describes a faintly sigmoid shape with steeper gradients in the early years and again before growth ceases than in the middle period (Figure 1.1a). These differences in the rate of growth are shown much more clearly by the velocity curve in which rate of growth, in centimetres per year, is expressed against age (Figure 1.1b). Postnatal growth can be seen to divide conveniently into three periods:

1. Infantile growth, a phase of rapid but decelerating growth, from birth until about two years of age, which represents an extrapolation of the prenatal growth curve.

2. Mid-childhood growth, a 'cruising' period of relatively constant growth from about two years to the start of the pubertal growth spurt. It is useful to remember that during this phase a growth rate consistently below about 5 cm per year is a cause for concern. In the short term, however, normal children may show remarkable variations in growth rate. These are often seasonal, some children growing twice as fast in the summer as in the winter. Normal children, especially boys, who enter puberty late may also have a very slow growth rate for some months before their growth spurt starts.

3. Pubertal growth, reached approximately two years earlier in girls than in boys, and consisting of a rapid acceleration in growth rate to a peak height velocity around 10 cm per year, then a symmetrical fall to zero as the epiphyses fuse and growth ceases. This period occupies about four and a half years.

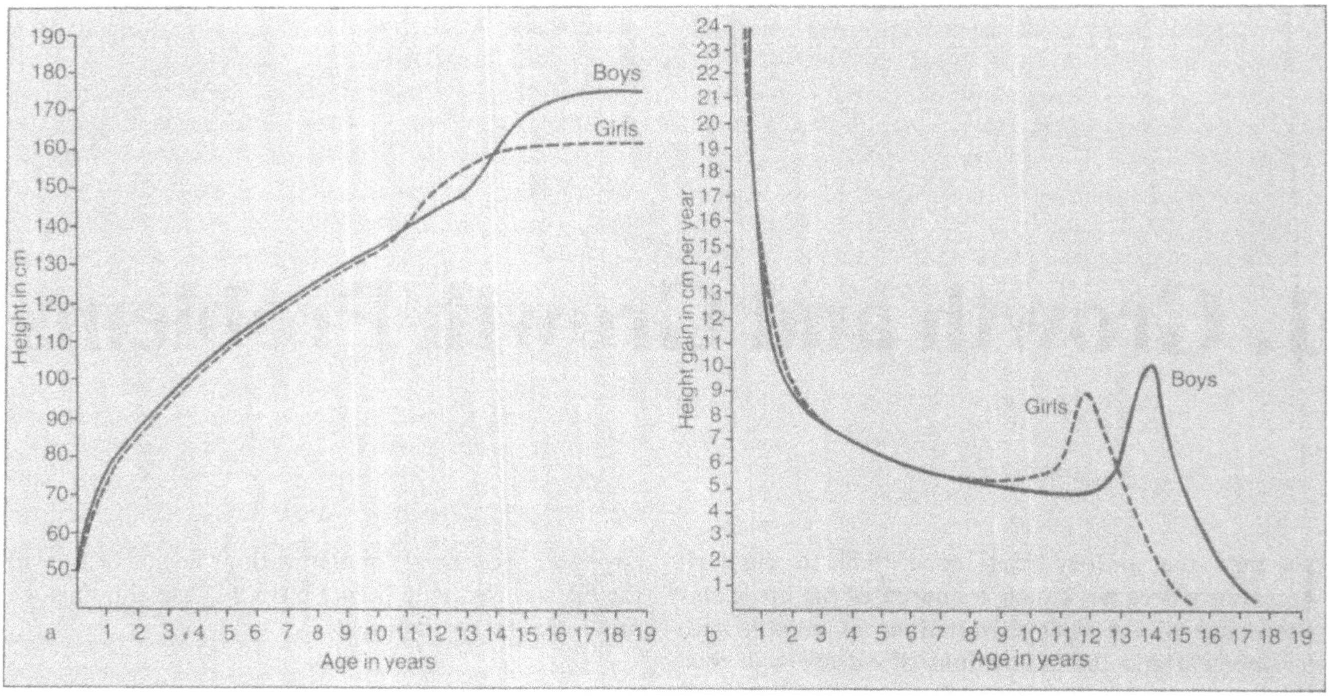

Figure 1.1. *Typical growth curves for boys and girls, a) height attained and b) growth velocity.*

Differential Growth

The general growth of the child conceals differential growth of great complexity. Measurement of height reflects changes in only one organ system, the skeleton, and different parts of this system are responsive to different influences and grow at different rates. At birth the head is large and the trunk and limbs short so that the upper to lower segment ratio is approximately 1.8:1.0. In mid-childhood, largely under the influence of growth hormone, the limbs grow relatively faster than the trunk so that by the start of puberty the ratio is 1:1. In contrast, pubertal growth, determined by adrenal and gonadal steroids, affects the trunk relatively more than the limbs (Figure 1.2). These differences account for the characteristic long limbs and 'eunuchoid' build of the late developer and the short limbs of the early developer.

There are greater differences in growth rate among different organ systems. The brain, for instance, is relatively mature at birth and has reached approximately 80 per cent of its adult size by two years; the lymphoid system attains its largest mass in mid-childhood and then starts to regress; the reproductive organs develop little after birth until puberty.

Rate of Maturation

An important concept in growth is that of 'maturational age'. The tempo of maturation varies considerably from one child to another. Some, with their 'clocks set fast', go through the whole process of development rapidly, while others, 'set slow', mature late and continue to grow until a relatively late age. There is a strong tendency for such patterns to be familial. Some means of estimating this aspect of development is vital in assessing growth problems. A rough indication of 'maturational' or 'physiological' age can be obtained clinically from dental development and, during puberty, from the development of the secondary sexual characteristics. Much the most useful indication, however, is the radiological bone age. This is assessed from an x-ray of the left wrist by comparing the maturity of the bones with suitable norms for the population.

Pubertal Development

The sequence of events at puberty in boys and girls is shown graphically in Figure 1.3. The Tanner system of staging is used and the details are given in Table 1.1. This system is widely accepted and forms an invaluable shorthand in dealing with problems of adolescent development. Many clinically useful points are apparent from Figure 1.3. Although girls are, on average, two years more mature than boys and their peak height velocity occurs two years earlier, the first sign of puberty—in girls this is usually breast development and in boys enlargement of the testes—occurs between the ages of 11 and 12 years in both sexes. Menarche is a relatively late event in female puberty and the height spurt is nearly complete by the time it occurs. Although,

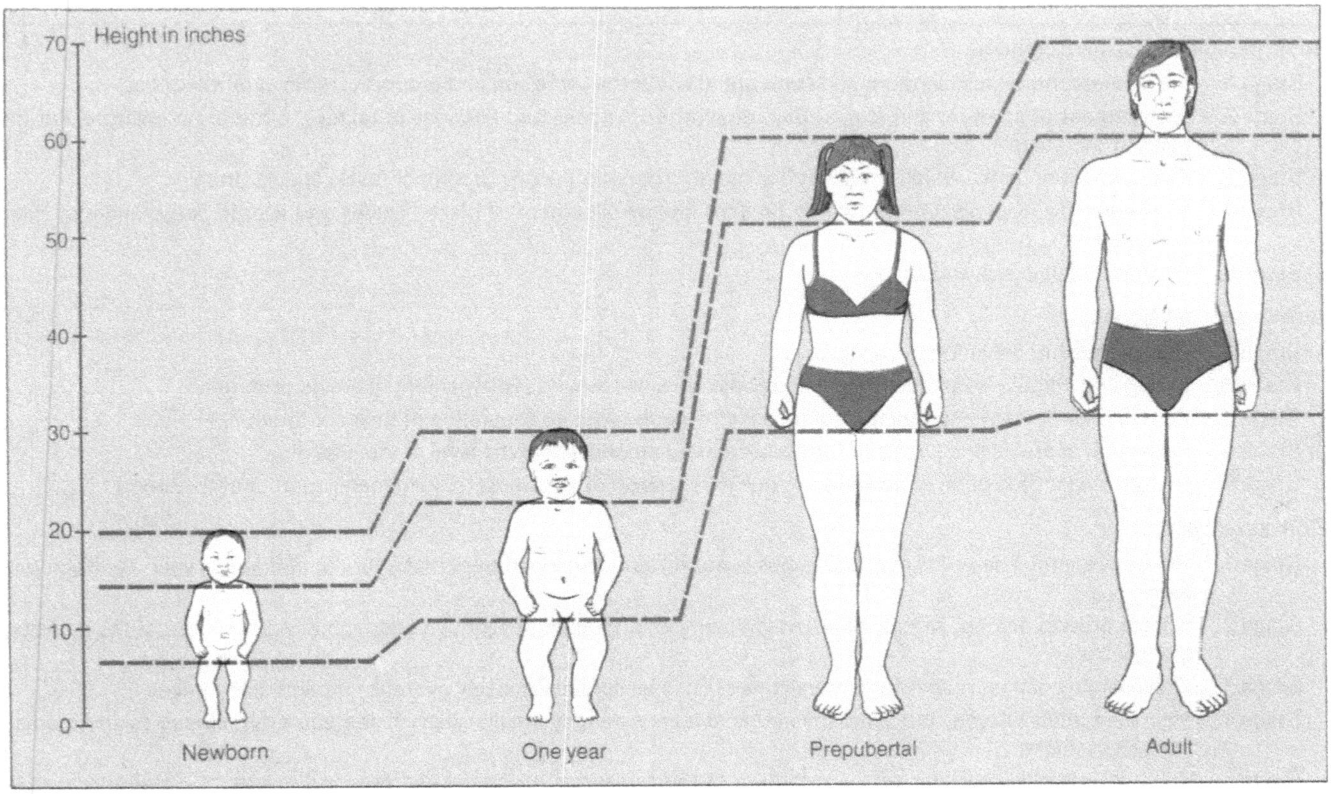

Figure 1.2. *Differential growth of the skeleton through childhood.*

in a secular trend, the age of menarche has gradually become younger in affluent populations over the last 200 years, evidence suggests that this trend has now ceased, with the average age of menarche at 13 years. The standard deviation of this, and indeed of most of the pubertal events defined, is approximately one year. It is simple, therefore, to remember that menarche before the age of 11 years or after the age of 15 years is more than two standard deviations displaced from the mean. The major events of puberty are now depicted on the Tanner-Whitehouse growth charts as centile bars (see Figures 1.8 and 1.9), a most useful addition.

Genetic Growth Potential

Growth is largely determined by genetic factors; there is, for instance, a high degree of correlation between the heights of identical twins. The height of each parent exerts an equal influence on the adult height of their children. It would obviously be unfortunate for small mothers if this held true for the dimensions of babies at birth, and in fact length and weight at birth are much more closely related to maternal size. Compensation for paternal size then occurs in the early months of life. This effect was graphically illustrated by experiments in which Shire horses were crossed with Shetland ponies! At birth the size of the foals reflected that of their

Figure 1.3. *The average timing of events at puberty for a) girls and b) boys. (See Table 1.1 for details.)*

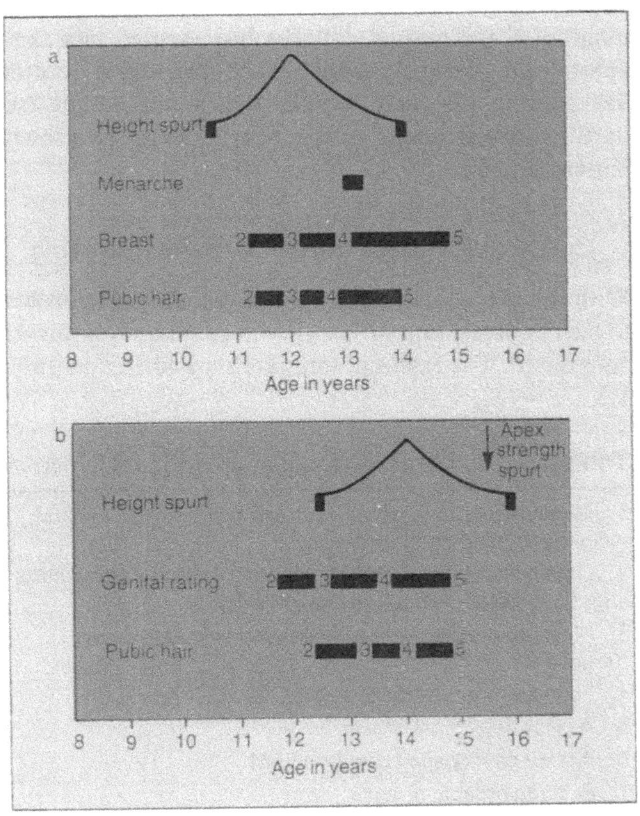

Table 1.1. The Tanner system of pubertal staging.

Boys: genital (penis) development:	
Stage 1.	Pre-adolescent: testes, scrotum and penis are of about the same size and proportion as in early childhood
Stage 2.	Enlargement of scrotum and testes. Skin of scrotum reddens and changes in texture. Little or no enlargement of penis at this stage
Stage 3.	Enlargement of penis, which occurs at first mainly in length. Further growth of testes and scrotum
Stage 4.	Increased size of penis with growth in breadth and development of glans. Testes and scotum larger; scrotal skin darkened
Stage 5.	Genitalia adult in size and shape
Girls: breast development:	
Stage 1.	Pre-adolescent: elevation of papilla only
Stage 2.	Breast bud stage: elevation of breast and papilla as small mound. Enlargement of areola diameter
Stage 3.	Further enlargement and elevation of breast and areola, with no separation of their contours
Stage 4.	Projection of areola and papilla to form a secondary mound above the level of the breast
Stage 5.	Mature stage: projection of papilla only, due to recession of the areola to the general contour of the breast
Both sexes: pubic hair:	
Stage 1.	Pre-adolescent. The vellus over the pubes is not further developed than that over the abdominal wall, i.e. no pubic hair
Stage 2.	Sparse growth of long, slightly pigmented downy hair, straight or slightly curled, chiefly at the base of the penis or along labia
Stage 3.	Considerably darker, coarser and more curled. The hair spreads sparsely over the junction of the pubes
Stage 4.	Hair now adult in type, but area covered is still considerably smaller than in the adult. No spread to the medial surface of thighs
Stage 5.	Adult in quantity and type with distribution of the horizontal (or classically 'feminine') pattern. Spread to medial surface of thighs but not up linea alba or elsewhere above the base of the inverse triangle (spread up linea alba occurs late and is rated stage 6)

mothers, but by two years of age the difference had largely disappeared (Figure 1.4). Similarly, by 18 months of age normal children have settled into their appropriate growth channels. The crossing of centile lines during the early months which this entails frequently leads to inappropriate worries about the growth pattern (Figure 1.5).

The Clinical Assessment of Growth Problems

With the preceding facts in mind, the clinical approach to a child presenting with a growth problem will now be considered. The essential steps are summarized in Table 1.2.

Table 1.2. Clinical assessment of growth problems.

1. Measure length (under 2 years) or height (over 2 years), weight and head circumference
2. Obtain all previous measurements, plot on growth charts and, if necessary, calculate growth velocity
3. Measure parents (and siblings) and calculate growth 'target area'
4. Estimate 'maturational' age
5. Assess nutritional intake
6. Assess psychosocial environment
7. Exclude organic disease

Measurement

Precise measurement of height in children is by no means easily achieved. Accurate measuring instruments (those illustrated in this chapter and used in most growth clinics in this country can be obtained from Holtain Ltd, of Crymmych, Pembrokeshire, UK) and consistent techniques are essential.

By convention supine length is measured until the age of two years. This requires two measurers, one to hold the infant's head firmly against the headboard and the other to grip the ankles, apply gentle traction and appose the foot board to the soles of the feet in the neutral position (Figure 1.6). After the age of two years, standing height is measured with the heels, back and head against a vertical surface. Light but firm stretching is essential to compensate for posture and the 'settling' effect which occurs through the day. This is achieved by applying upward pressure under the mastoid processes with the head in the neutral position while a counter-balanced head board is allowed to rest on the vertex (Figure 1.7). Sitting height, the most reproducible measure of trunk height, can be measured similarly with the child sitting on a flat surface of known height. Given these conditions and a single observer, measurements of great accuracy can be made. Unfortunately, the in-accuracy of the instruments available in most clinics and

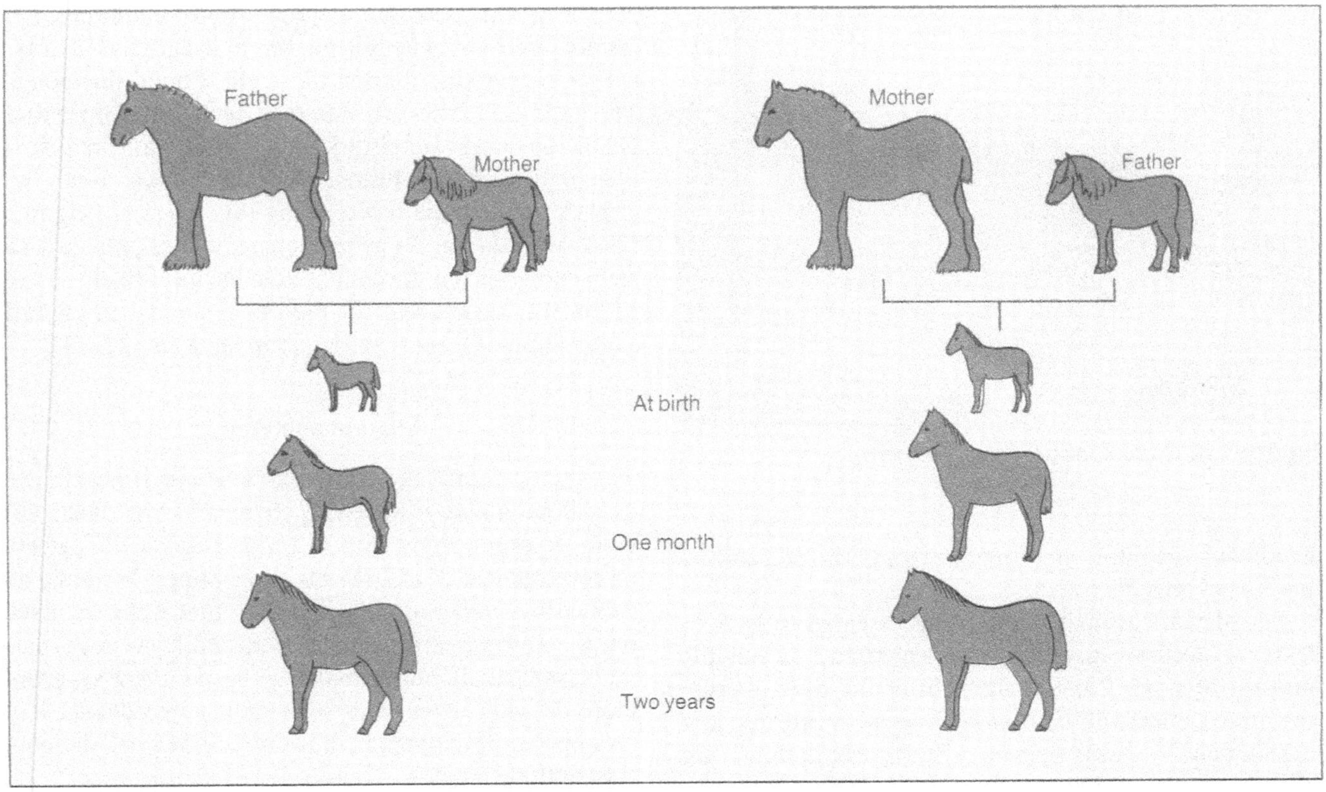

Figure 1.4. *The effect of parental size on the offspring of Shire horse by Shetland pony crosses.*

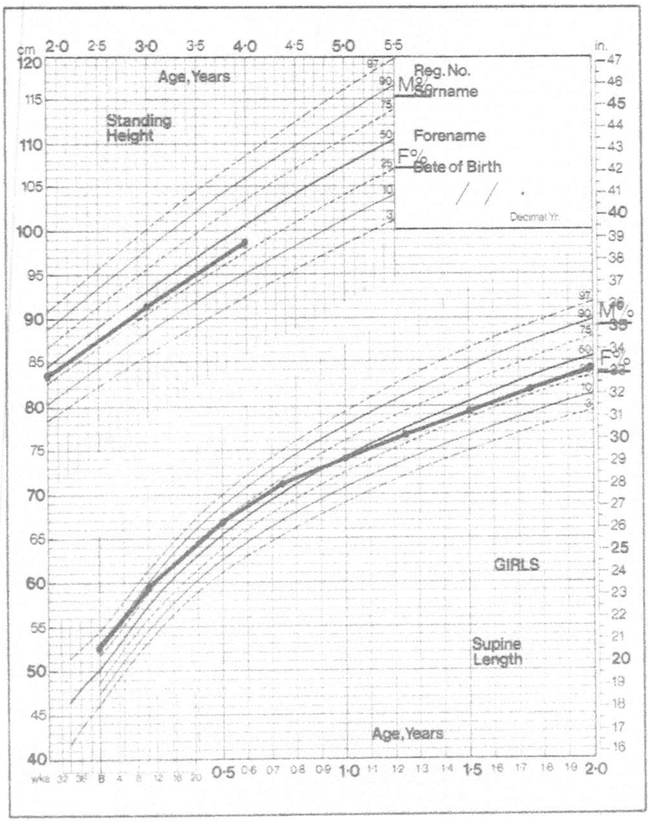

Figure 1.5. *The growth chart of a child of a relatively tall mother and short father. Although on the 80th centile for length at birth, by the age of 18 months her growth had settled around the 30th centile.*

surgeries and the errors of different observers often render measurements useless.

The measurements obtained should be plotted on suitable growth charts. These must be representative of the population from which the child is drawn. The Tanner–Whitehouse charts (obtainable from Castlemead Publications Ltd, Hertford SG14 1LH, UK) are the best available for British children and are illustrated in this chapter. Since body proportions are, in the statistical sense, normally distributed, growth charts are able to indicate not only the mean but also the range of measurements at a given age by displaying standard deviations or centiles (the 50th centile representing the mean, and the 97th and third approximately plus and minus two standard deviations). The further any measurement lies from the mean the more likely it is to be abnormal but it is important to remember that, by definition, three per cent of the normal population fall below the third and three per cent fall above the 97th centile.

Previous Measurements

In assessing any aspect of growth the most important single fact is the rate of change. However far from the population mean the height of a child may be, investigation will not prove rewarding if the current rate of growth is normal. Conversely, if a child is of average

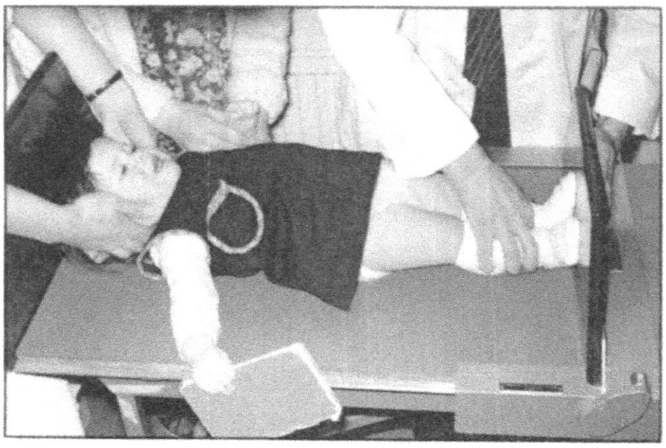

Figure 1.6. *Supine length measurement.*

height for age but is growing too slowly or too rapidly, the reason must be sought.

To calculate growth velocity it is essential to have at least two accurate measurements separated by a suitable interval of time. Clearly, the shorter the time interval the more critical will be changes in growth rate and any inaccuracy in measurement. Such calculations are greatly simplified by the use of the 'decimal year' in which each day is expressed as a decimal of the whole year. A table indicating the decimal value of each day of the year is printed on the back of the Tanner-Whitehouse growth charts. Time elapsed is expressed as a decimal and growth velocity calculated as:

$$\frac{\text{change in height}}{\text{time elapsed}}$$

If, for instance, a child measured 106.3 cm on 3 March 1979 (decimal = 79.17) and 111.7 cm on 6 June 1980 (decimal = 80.43) his average growth velocity through this period was:

$$\frac{111.7-106.3}{80.43-79.17} = 4.3 \text{ cm/yr}$$

Observation for at least one full year is necessary for definitive conclusions to be drawn, but with accurate measurement three-month periods give a useful indication of growth rate.

Parental Heights

The child's parents should, if possible, be measured, since even their own estimates of their heights may be remarkably inaccurate. With the parental heights it is possible to make an estimate of the genetic height expectation of the child. This is most easily done by using the 'mid-parental centile'. This is the midpoint between the height centiles of the parents, which are read off from appropriate sex growth charts and entered on the child's chart. Since the height of each parent has an equal effect on the adult height of the child, the mean height of the potential population of children of a certain marriage will fall on the mid-parental centile, with a normal distribution of height around this point. The band enclosing two standard deviations above and below the mean extends 8.5 cm above and 8.5 cm below this point and has been called the 'target area' for growth. If the band representing this range of height is filled in on the child's growth chart, it is usually easy to see whether or not the child's final height is likely to fall within the target area, see Figures 1.8 and 1.9. (A full explanation of these two figures appears on page 13.)

Maturational Age

The maturational age should be assessed from clinical examination and, if necessary, from an x-ray of the left wrist. It is important also to enquire about the pattern of development of the parents and siblings. Virtually all women remember at what age their menarche occurred but the absence of an equally memorable event in male adolescent development makes retrospective assessment more difficult. Men who were unusually advanced or retarded in development, however, remember the contrast with their peers.

Psychosocial Environment

It is a remarkable but incontrovertible fact that many children reared in an adverse psychosocial environment fail to grow normally, even when they are offered an

Figure 1.7. *Standing height measurement.*

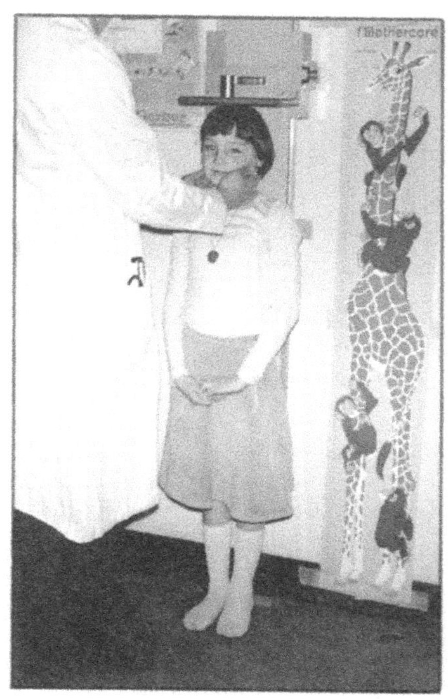

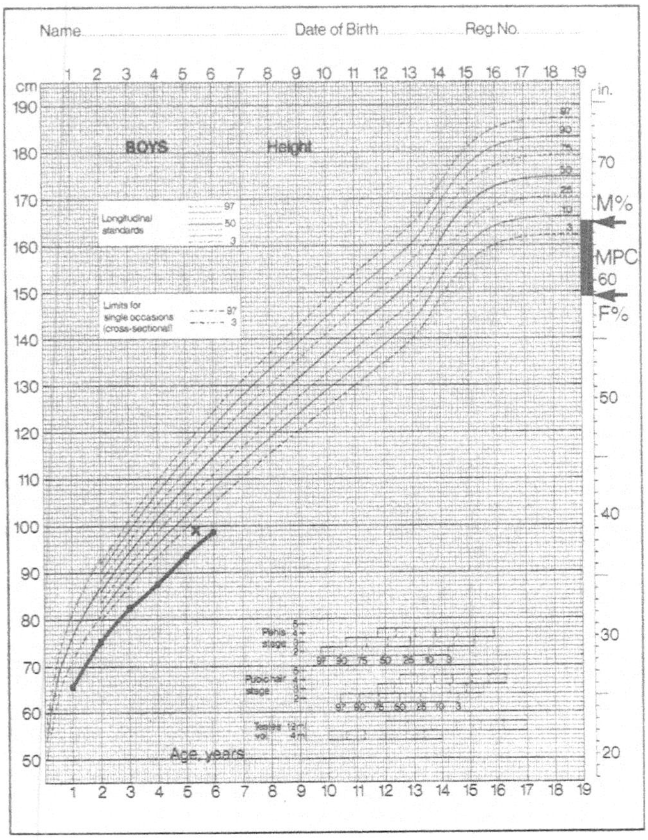

Figure 1.8. *The growth chart of a genetically short child. The bone age is indicated by a cross and the 'target area' (see text) is shaded.*

entirely adequate diet (see Figure 1.10). It is most important, therefore, to make a preliminary assessment of the environment of any child presenting with unexplained growth retardation. If there is any suspicion that environmental factors may be important, psychosocial evaluation should be undertaken before any other form of investigation, to save the child investigations which are not only unnecessary but may give misleading results.

Organic Disease

Although any illness may affect growth, only relatively few conditions regularly present with disturbance of growth as a primary feature. In the obligatory full general history and physical examination of a child with a growth problem, therefore, special attention must be paid to any indication of endocrine, metabolic, malabsorptive, renal and other relatively 'silent' problems.

Problems of Growth in Infancy—'Failure to Thrive'

'Failure to thrive' is a well established cliché for one of the commonest paediatric problems—inadequate weight gain and/or linear growth in infancy. With its overtones of horticulture and veterinary medicine, failure to thrive is not a term of which we are especially fond, but paediatrics has more than a little in common with these disciplines and perhaps it is salutary to be reminded of the similarities between the growth problems of babies, seedlings and piglets!

A basic axiom of paediatrics states that all serious illness will affect growth and that the more rapid the growth rate the more pronounced this effect will be. It has already been emphasized that postnatal growth velocity is at a maximum during infancy, not only in terms of weight gain and linear growth but also brain growth, reflected in clinical measurement by the head circumference. Infants are therefore uniquely vulnerable to conditions which disturb general somatic growth and also brain growth and the problem of failure to thrive requires rapid and thorough evaluation.

It is a fortunate fact that, as every general practitioner is well aware, only a small minority of children presenting in this way prove to have significant organic illness. This is true at all stages of the referral process, which often progresses from mother to father to grand-

Figure 1.9. *Delayed growth and maturation in one of two sisters. Bone ages at different chronological ages are indicated with crosses and show consistent retardation. M indicates menarche. The 'target area' (see text) is shaded.*

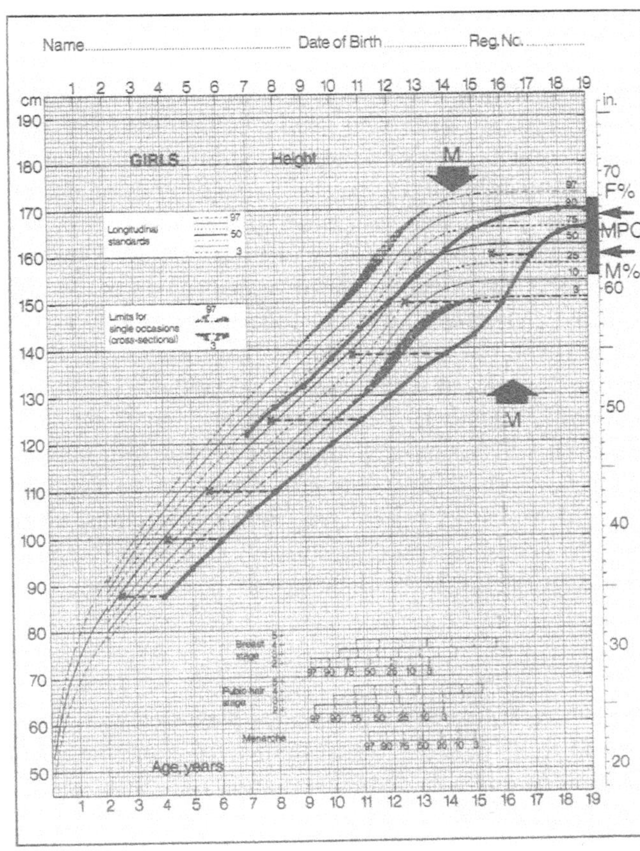

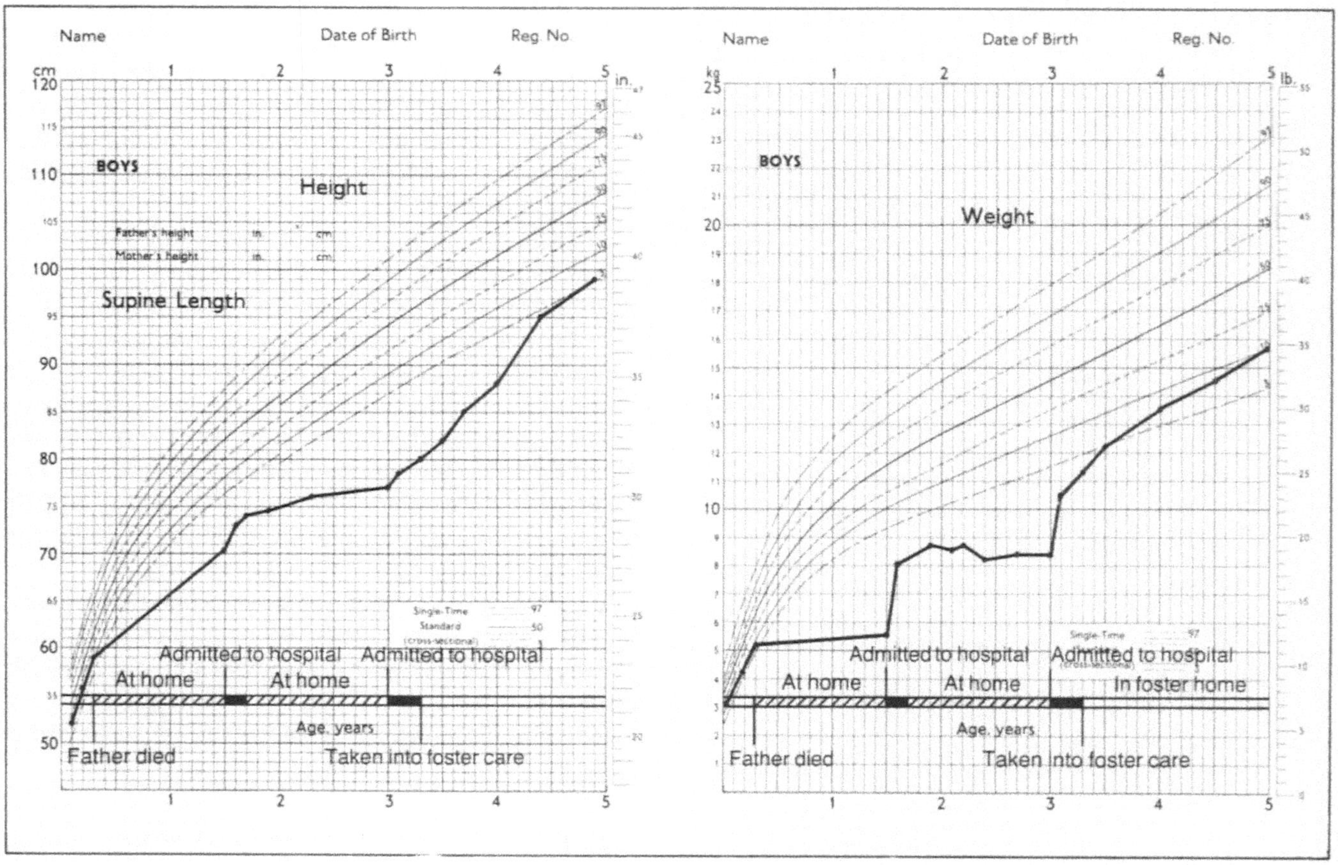

Figure 1.10. *The growth chart of a child who suffered severe deprivation, both emotional and nutritional, after his father died. Note the remarkable growth acceleration after admission to hospital and the rapid catch-up growth which occurred when he was taken into foster care.*

mother to neighbour to local grand multipara to health visitor and to well baby clinic before reaching the general practitioner, and then, exceptionally, passing to the paediatrician! Even for those standing, as we do, at the end of this line, a major function is simple reassurance and re-education of the mother. Thus in our alliterative classification of the major causes of failure to thrive in Table 1.3 we conclude far more often that the problem lies among the first five 'functional' than among the second five organic categories. The main diagnostic dilemma is therefore to sort out those situations in which simple advice and support are needed from those in which investigation must be thoroughly pursued. (It is, of course, in just these circumstances that the doctor can most easily, although inadvertently, cause anxiety rather than relieve it.)

Clinical Assessment

The clinical information required to assess growth problems in infancy is essentially similar to that for older children (Table 1.2) but differs in detail. A rigid approach is unlikely to be rewarded and, as always in paediatrics, it is necessary to be flexible and opportunistic in gathering clinical information, both historical from relatives and physical from the infant. Some amplification of the steps given in Table 1.2 may be useful.

Measurement

The basic measurements are weight, length and head circumference. With satisfactory apparatus and careful technique, accurate weighing should be simple but errors occur frequently. The measurement of length (described on page 4) is difficult even for trained observers with good apparatus. If a specially constructed table is not available a reasonably accurate length can be obtained using any firm, flat surface apposed to a wall. As described, the head of the infant is held firmly against the wall by one measurer while the other holds both ankles in one hand, lightly stretches the child and brings a right-angled object into contact with the soles of the feet in the neutral position. The measurement is then marked, the infant removed and his length measured with a tape. (Crown–rump length, measured with the hips fully flexed, is equivalent to sitting height in older children.) However, because

Table 1.3. Major causes of failure to thrive.

Misconceptions	Genetic small size
	Normal growth variation
	Premature and small for dates infants
Mistakes	Incorrect weighing or measurement
	Underfeeding
	Incorrect or wrongly constituted feeds
Misgivings	Maternal (or medical) lack of confidence
Misery	Crying infant
	Maternal depression
Mishandling	Child abuse
	Neglect
Malabsorption	Cystic fibrosis
	Coeliac disease
	Carbohydrate intolerance
	Milk protein intolerance
Microbes	Urinary tract infection
	Chest infection
	Enteritis
	Congenital infection
Malformations	Dysmorphic syndromes
	Genetic and chromosomal disorders
	Cardiac, renal tract, gut, CNS malformations
Metabolic	Hypothyroidism, hypopituitarism
	Hypercalcaemia
	Renal tubular acidosis, nephrogenic diabetes insipidus
Malignancy	CNS
	Intra-abdominal

accurate measurement of length poses such problems and because head circumference reflects the growth of the brain, this measurement is of equal or greater importance in early life. Head circumference measurement also holds pitfalls for the unwary, such as stretched cloth tapes, and interobserver variation is considerable.

Previous Measurements

Infants are the only children for whom previous measurements are usually available. Birth weight is always recorded and almost always remembered accurately by the mother. Birth length too is usually recorded but often represents little more than a guess by the midwife. Birth head circumference measurement tends to be more accurate and can usually be obtained from the neonatal record. Postnatal measurements seldom comprise more than the well baby clinic weight record, but this is often a most useful document to consult.

In the infant, as in the older child, the importance of growth velocity and genetic expectation cannot be overemphasized. A frequent cause for anxiety, for instance, is an unusually small or large head. Such a feature is likely to be a normal genetic variation but can be of the greatest clinical importance if it reflects a serious remediable problem, such as craniostenosis or hydrocephalus. Essential information includes parental head size, because genetic factors are no less important in head than in general somatic size, and the rate of growth. Head growth velocity charts are available but it is generally adequate to plot sequential measurements carefully on a growth chart and to judge by eye whether the gradient is deviating from an acceptable velocity. The Gairdner chart (Figure 1.11), on which infantile length, weight and head circumference centiles are displayed, is particularly useful for this purpose.

In one important aspect, however, infants differ from older children because deviation from a 'growth channel' along a centile line is much less likely to indicate disease. Many infants cross centile lines in the early months of life while settling into the growth channel appropriate for their genetic growth potential and maturational rate (see Figure 1.5).

Assessment of Nutritional Intake

Misconceptions concerning feeding still abound and growth failure due to inadequate energy intake is remarkably common. It is usually a straightforward matter to establish with reasonable accuracy what a

Figure 1.11. *Height, weight and head circumference centiles for boys aged 0–2 years. (Gairdner chart.)*

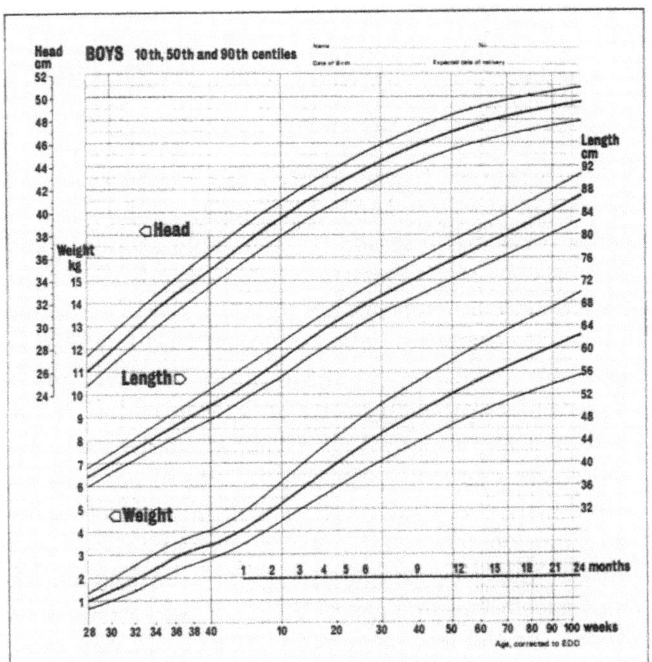

bottle fed infant is receiving, but this cannot be done for the breast fed infant without the laborious, and often lactation-inhibiting, process of test weighing. One of the few problems following in the wake of the recent welcome emphasis on the benefits of the breast has been the increase in the number of infants who are victims of well-intentioned starvation.

Assessment of Psychosocial Environment

The overwhelming importance of the maternal-child relationship, not only in emotional but also in physical development, is well established. The infant is a dependent being who relies very largely on one individual for food, care, love and stimulation. It is hardly surprising, therefore, that serious physical, psychological or social problems affecting the mother or mother-substitute have a profound effect on the dependent member of this unique relationship (see Figure 1.10).

Exclusion of Organic Disease

A systematic history is likely to provide the first indication of underlying disease in infants with organic problems. The physical examination must include a thorough search for stigmata of congenital abnormality and signs of disease in any system, and note must be taken of the nonspecific signs which may accompany growth failure, such as dehydration, wasting, delayed closure of the fontanelles and failure of the teeth to erupt. Examination of the urine should perhaps be included in the routine physical examination because it is so easily omitted in infants and yet frequently provides the only clue to serious renal problems.

Major Causes of Failure to Thrive (Table 1.3)

Misconceptions

Misconceptions remain remarkably widespread. The most common is inappropriate anxiety about a small infant when the reason is apparent, such as small parental size, racial variation (centile charts for English children are not appropriate for other races: the infants of parents from the Indian continent and Far East are generally smaller), prematurity or low birth weight for dates. It is more difficult to assess the growth of infants who are, as mentioned above, crossing channels. This pattern is frequently observed in infants who are relatively large or small at birth and doubt is resolved by a period of observation (Figure 1.5). Normal variations in weight gain frequently cause anxiety in mothers who may have been led to expect that their baby will gain one ounce, or the less memorable 30 g, every day except Sundays!

Mistakes

The simplest mistakes arise as a result of errors in measurement, and often lead to unnecessary anxiety. More important are the errors leading to inadequate or inappropriate feeding of the infant. These frequently arise from over-rigid ideas on the timing (a four-hourly schedule was not decreed in heaven and is inappropriate for many small infants) or quantity of feeds (the same applies to the magic 2.5 oz/lb or 170 ml/kg!). As the baby milks are improved and their reconstitution is simplified and standardized, errors arising from the composition and concentration of the milk are fortunately becoming much less common, but they remain an important cause of difficulty.

Misgivings and Misery

Although there are now sources of sound advice available to the young mother she may feel insecure and afraid and find it difficult to make use of them. Postnatal depression is often a factor in these difficulties and such mothers require much support through the early weeks. The tendency, however, always to ascribe difficult behaviour in the infant to insecurity or incompetence in the mother is unfortunate. There is no doubt that some infants are more irritable and demanding than others and the mother of such an infant should be reminded of this fact and told that irritable infants do not necessarily become irritable children and adults! She may further appreciate assurance that the feelings of overwhelming and saintly maternal love for her infant which she was led to expect may be severely strained by resentment of this dependent, demanding and ungrateful little person.

Mishandling

Sadly, all involved with children should now be acutely aware of the dangers of frank child abuse (see Chapter 17), especially by parents who were themselves deprived and often maltreated. Here the background knowledge of the general practitioner concerning the family may be of the greatest value, but all doctors must be sensitive to the various appeals for help which can be channelled through complaints about an infant's progress. Passive neglect is even more common than active abuse and can be as damaging to the child.

Microbes

A history of nonspecific ill-health and growth failure raises the possibility of covert infection. The most frequent site is the renal tract and the importance of urine testing, including microscopy and culture, has already been emphasized. In virtually all cases of chronic pyelonephritis the damage to the kidneys has started in infancy. Fortunately, most other chronic bacterial infections are now rare but tuberculosis, especially in immigrants, must not be forgotten. The symptoms of pertussis may drag on for many weeks and affected infants frequently lose much weight. Recurrent chest infections, especially with staphylococci, raise the possibility of fibrocystic disease. Persistent gut infections and infestations, e.g. with pathogenic *E. coli*, *Salmonella* or *Giardia*, may affect weight gain without obvious diarrhoea. Prenatally acquired infection, such as rubella, toxoplasmosis, cytomegalovirus and syphilis, may be associated with severe failure to thrive as well as more specific problems. The possibility of immunodeficiency should be considered in an infant who suffers either an excessive number of infections or seems prone to infection with organisms of low virulence.

Malabsorption

In contrast to many of the other disorders which may present as failure to thrive, malabsorption is possibly more often suspected than present. Fibrocystic disease, which has an incidence of approximately 1 in 2,000, may present in this way and must be excluded in any infant who fails to grow adequately in spite of a normal, or indeed large, intake, whether or not there are associated pulmonary problems. Coeliac disease, which is now frequently diagnosed in the first year of life (Figure 1.12), is generally associated with less prominent gastrointestinal symptoms but marked growth failure. The relationship of the symptoms to the introduction of cereal into the diet is seldom obvious. Intolerance of disaccharide sugars often follows a gastrointestinal insult, such as surgery or gastroenteritis, and causes diarrhoea with loose, acid, irritant and often frothy stools. Reducing substances can be detected in the stool supernatant with Clinitest tablets. Allergy to cows' milk is increasingly recognized and may present with gastrointestinal symptoms and failure to thrive.

Malformations

Congenital abnormalities of many types may be associated with growth failure. It is a prime feature of the major genetic abnormalities, such as the trisomies and Turner's syndrome, and indeed is prominent, although seldom the presenting feature, in most dysmorphic syndromes. Malformations of single organ systems, e.g. congenital heart disease, especially when cyanotic, and cerebral malformations, are also associated with growth failure. Renal tract malformations may lead to renal failure or predispose to infection. Gastrointestinal malformations may result in failure to thrive from feeding difficulties, vomiting or diarrhoea, or malabsorption.

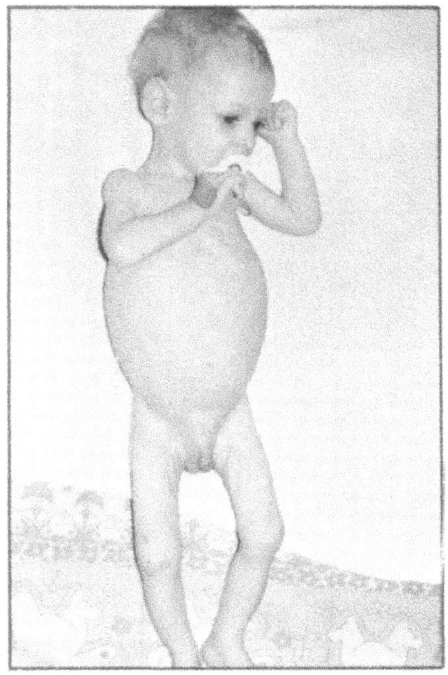

Figure 1.12. *An infant, aged 9 months, with coeliac disease showing the characteristic pallor, wasting, distended abdomen and sad expression.*

Metabolic Disturbances

Many metabolic disturbances are associated with prominent growth failure (Figure 1.13). It is the cardinal feature of hypothyroidism (Figure 1.14) and growth hormone deficiency, conditions which, although rare, are eminently amenable to treatment (see pages 15-16).

Malignancy

Tumours are rare in infancy. Most arise in the CNS or intra-abdominal organs. They may present with non-specific symptoms of failure to thrive and, as early treatment may be curative, they must be considered in the differential diagnosis of obscure growth failure.

Management of Failure to Thrive

Growth Normal

Once satisfied that there is no real growth problem it may be, and often is, a straightforward matter to provide the information and reassurance needed. The centile charts are often most helpful in convincing parents that growth is normal. When this proves more difficult than it should, however, the prudent general practitioner will ask himself whether the apparent anxiety about growth may have concealed other unexpressed fears about the baby.

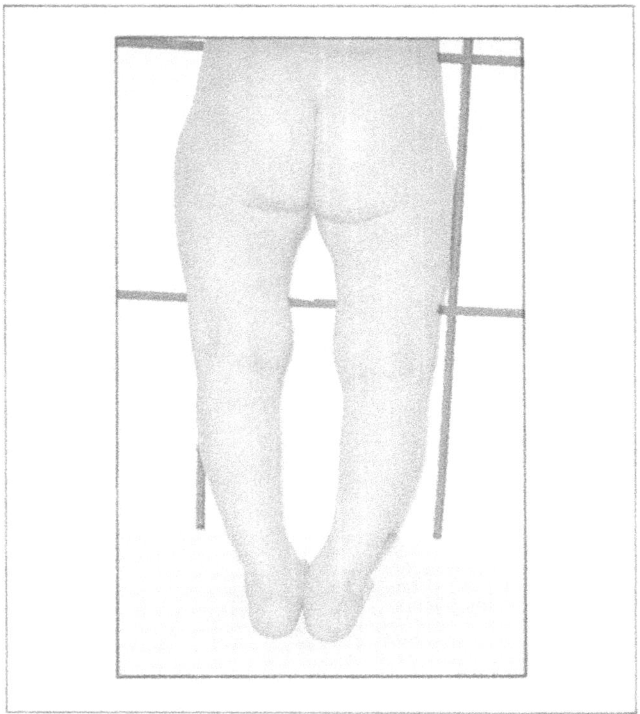

Figure 1.13. *The legs of a two-year-old child whose growth failure proved to be due to familial hypophosphataemic rickets.*

Figure 1.14. *A hypothyroid infant, aged 22 months, who presented with growth failure in spite of good weight gain. He shows the characteristic facies, plump build and short limbs.*

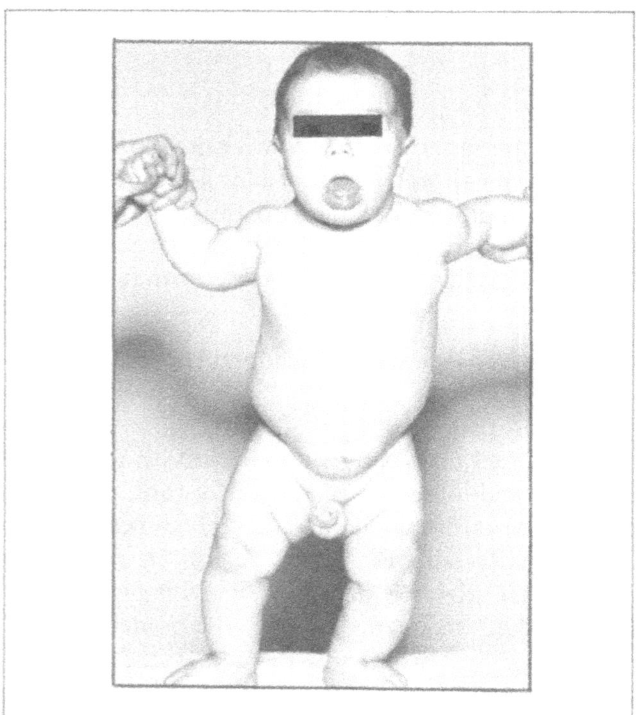

Not Sure

Frequently the only possible verdict, especially after the first consultation, will be the Scottish 'not proven'. We find, however, that we can usually subdivide this category into two parts—the 'probably normals' and the 'probably abnormals'.

Probably normal. These are the infants about whom some doubt remains, usually because of lack of sufficient measurements to assess growth rate. Reassurance and arrangements to make further measurements after a suitable interval are generally all that is needed.

Probably abnormal. When the index of suspicion is higher but doubt still remains, it may be appropriate to conduct a number of simple screening investigations before or during a period of close observation.

Growth Abnormal

This category also may be subdivided as follows.

Cause apparent, in which case appropriate management can be instituted immediately.

Cause not apparent, in which case investigation must be pursued until the reason for the growth failure is clear. If necessary enlist the services of your local paediatrician.

Growth Problems in Older Children

Growth problems come in two sizes, too small and too tall. The terms short and tall stature are preferred to 'dwarfism' and 'gigantism' because these, especially in the minds of children, are strongly associated with magic, mystery and mischief!

Short Stature

Short stature has dual importance: not only do most children, especially boys, find their lack of height distressing but failure to grow may indicate serious underlying disease. A simplified classification of the causes of growth retardation is presented in Table 1.4.

Genetic Short Stature

Small parents beget small children. They are usually well aware of this biological fact but many find it difficult to accept, especially if their size has been a cause of distress to them. It is painful for parents to watch their children suffering the same agonies that they themselves experienced. Many such couples therefore seek assurance that their small child is simply following the family pattern and that no treatment can help. When the clinical information specified in Table 1.4 has

Table 1.4. Causes of short stature.

Genetic short stature
Delayed maturation
Prenatal growth retardation
Chromosome anomalies
Psychosocial growth retardation
Malnutrition
Skeletal disorders
Systemic disease
Endocrine disorders

been obtained, it is usually apparent that the child's growth is normal. Figure 1.8 (page 7) shows the growth chart of such a child. His father was exceptionally short but fully fit and his mother a small normal woman. The social circumstances were satisfactory and physical examination was normal. His growth curve between the ages of one and six years showed that, although he was well below the third centile in height, he had maintained his position parallel to it. His bone age was $5\frac{1}{4}$ years at a chronological age of six, a disparity which is within normal limits. Extrapolation of his growth curve showed that he was likely to fall well within the 'target area' calculated from the mid-parental centile. His parents were assured that no form of treatment could enhance his growth potential. Such families are especially common in centres of the horse-racing community such as that included in the authors' area of practice!

Delayed Maturation

Simple maturational delay is common and, since such children may be very small in comparison with their peers, it often causes anxiety. Because of the strong tendency for the problem to be familial, it is reassuring if another member of the family has shown a similar pattern of development. Additional clues include delay in dental and/or pubertal development and significant retardation of the bone age in the absence of any other abnormality.

The children about whom there is most likely to be anxiety are those in whom delay is associated with familial short stature. Children destined to be of average or tall height, even if they are delayed in maturation, are unlikely to be really short in childhood. Many such children, however, present in the pubertal years when all their friends overtake them in height and development. The growth curves of two sisters are depicted in Figure 1.9 (page 7). Their mother had not started her periods until the age of 16. The older girl was average in growth and only slightly delayed in development compared with her peers but the younger was very small throughout her childhood and fell much further behind when her friends went into puberty. However, as predicted, she eventually achieved a height only a little shorter than her sister and well within the parental 'target area'. No investigation other than monitoring of her growth and bone age was undertaken and, suitably reassured and possessed of a cheerful and optimistic personality, she was able to make capital of her years as the smallest girl in the class, protected by all and permitted licence denied to her larger and more mature peers!

The problem of delayed maturation presents the doctor with two main dilemmas. The first is to exclude organic disease of the hypothalamic-pituitary-gonadal axis or of any other system; investigation must not be too long delayed in children with atypical findings or severe degrees of retardation. The second is to decide whether to offer more active treatment in those children without organic problems, in whom careful explanation and reassurance seem insufficient. This is occasionally justified, especially in children whose height potential is good so that the loss of a small amount of final height will be of little consequence. Anabolic steroids in low doses can induce considerable acceleration in growth rate without virilization in prepubertal children, but the acceleration in skeletal maturity may be greater than that in growth so final height may be compromised. During puberty, growth and sexual development may be accelerated in boys by testosterone and, to a lesser extent, in girls by oestrogen. This form of treatment may be of real psychological benefit in boys with significant delay but it should be closely monitored, and we would recommend that it is undertaken only under the supervision of a growth clinic.

Prenatal Growth Retardation

Prenatal growth retardation may result from many causes including placental insufficiency, inherited disorders, chromosomal abnormalities, intrauterine infections and maternal exposure to smoking, alcohol or drugs, but in the majority of infants who are short or light for dates no cause is apparent. Some infants, such as twins whose growth retardation was caused by uterine constraint, show rapid catch-up growth in the early months of life. Those with severe prenatal growth retardation, however, seldom show more than a slight and gradual tendency to catch up.

In addition to low birth length and weight, some children with idiopathic prenatal growth retardation show characteristic physical features including asymmetry of one side of the body compared with the other, a lack of fat, a characteristic facial appearance with a relatively large vault and small triangular face with down-turned 'shark' mouth, and incurved little fingers. Several syndromes have been defined, such as those of Silver and Russell, but these have failed to subdivide this group of children usefully, and it seems preferable to lump them together under the heading of prenatal growth retardation until specific causes can be found. Such children usually have growth curves below but parallel to the third centile lines.

Chromosomal Abnormalities

With the exceptions mentioned under Tall Stature (page 17), children with major chromosomal abnormalities are almost invariably short but many, such as those with the trisomies, have multiple morphological problems which cause more immediate concern than their lack of stature.

The chromosomal anomaly most likely to present as short stature, and always to be considered in short girls, is Turner's syndrome. Classically, the genotype is monosomic for the X chromosome, 45 XO, and so can be detected by absence of Barr bodies in a buccal smear, but many girls with a similar phenotype show mosaic patterns, with normal XX as well as XO cell lines, or abnormalities of one X chromosome. Studies of spontaneous abortions show that, like other monosomies, the XO phenotype is frequently lethal but it is unique in the fact that a significant proportion of affected fetuses do survive. Turner's syndrome and its variants are surprisingly common: the incidence is approximately one in 3,000 live births. A karyotype should therefore be requested in every girl with unexplained short stature.

The phenotypic features of the condition are protean and are generally more fully expressed in those with the XO genotype (Figure 1.15). Short stature is universal but the degree reflects parental height. Ovarian dysgenesis with lack or absence of germinal follicles occurs in more than 90 per cent, and other frequent anomalies include congenital lymphoedema, sometimes transient, of the dorsum of the hands and feet (approximately 80 per cent), 'shield' chest with widely spaced hypoplastic nipples (80 per cent), anomalies of the face and external ears and a low posterior hairline (80 per cent), cubitus valgus (70 per cent), hypoplastic finger and toenails (70 per cent) and renal anomalies (50 per cent). About 20 per cent show cardiac defects of which coarctation of the aorta is most common. Mental retardation, contrary to popular belief, is uncommon, occurring in only about 10 per cent of patients.

The management of Turner's syndrome requires full explanation to the parents and also to the child in relation to her level of understanding. Anabolic steroids may have a small part to play in promoting growth in childhood. At the age of puberty oestrogen replacement is needed to induce breast development and, since cyclical treatment is necessary to ensure shedding of the endometrium, this can conveniently be given in the form of one of the combined contraceptive preparations.

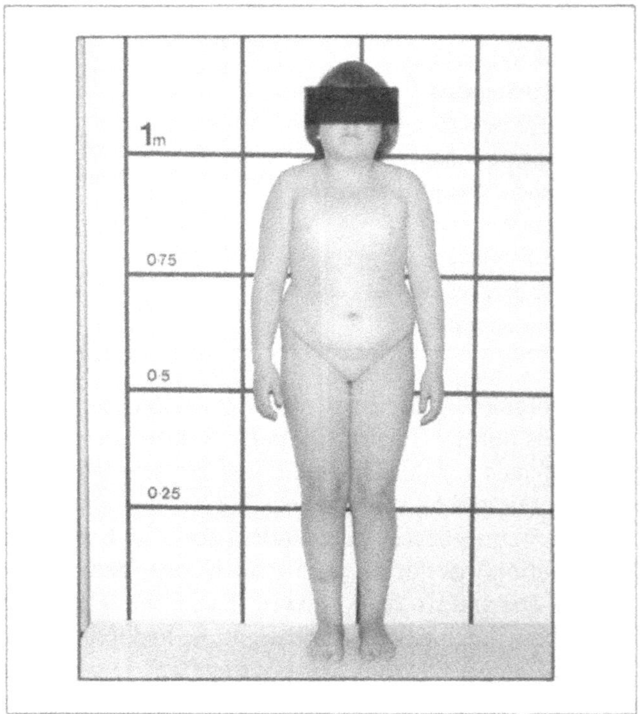

Figure 1.15. *A 12-year-old girl with XO Turner's syndrome. Note her short stature, lack of sexual development, 'square' build, short (but not obviously webbed) neck and 'shield' chest.*

Psychosocial Growth Retardation

Children in inhospitable psychosocial environments may fail to grow normally even though their caloric requirements are amply supplied. The pathophysiology of this phenomenon is obscure but it seems to be related, at least in part, to a switching off of growth hormone secretion. In practice, of course, children in deprived environments are often the victims of a variety of adverse circumstances, including low genetic height expectation, poor maternal nutrition through pregnancy and an inadequate or unbalanced diet, in addition to lack of stimulation and emotional warmth. Failure to grow is certainly one of the more subtle indications of the cycle of deprivation, and population studies have shown that such factors are among the most common causes of short stature in the community (Lacey and Parkin 1974). Similarly, psychosocial failure to thrive in infants is increasingly recognized to be an important indicator of child abuse. Doctors must be aware of this entity because the history obtained in the surgery or clinic is unlikely to reveal more than subtle clues to the degree of deprivation to which the child is subject. The growth retardation is almost invariably accompanied by behavioural disturbance and, indeed, this is often the presenting feature. Most characteristic is disturbance of appetite which may amount to an obsession with food, such children often eating excessively and stealing food whenever possible. Temper tantrums and negative behaviour are also common and the child's developmental progress may show considerable delay. Bulky and offensive stools may be another complaint.

Clinically, the growth failure may be indistinguishable from that of growth hormone deficiency or coeliac disease, with proportionate small stature and delay in skeletal maturation. The results of investigations may also be extremely difficult to differentiate from growth hormone deficiency or malabsorption, and the diagnosis can be confirmed finally only by observing improved growth and development after removal to a suitable environment. Full mobilization of community and medical resources to assist the family will sometimes correct the problem but in extreme cases the only solution is to remove the child into care.

Malnutrition

Uncomplicated malnutrition of sufficient severity to cause serious growth retardation is uncommon in our society, but is the most frequent cause of growth retardation in the chronically undernourished majority of the world's population. The problem is most serious in infancy, when not only general physical growth but also brain growth is at its most rapid, and more than 100 calories and 2 to 3 g of protein per kg of body weight are needed daily for optimal development.

In a generally overfed community, malnutrition may also crop up in less obvious contexts. These include breast fed infants with failure to thrive, children of parents with food fads, and adolescent girls with borderline anorexia nervosa, all of whom may suffer undernutrition of sufficient severity to impede growth.

Skeletal Disorders

The osteochondrodystrophies are a complex group of familial disorders. The effects on growth may be gross or extremely subtle. The chief diagnostic clue to such disorders is the fact that the growth failure is disproportionate, either with relatively long limbs and a short trunk, as in the spondyloepiphysial dysplasias (Figure 1.16) or short limbs and a relatively long trunk, as in achondroplasia and related conditions. In few such conditions is the biochemical abnormality yet understood so the diagnosis is largely radiological. Although no treatment is likely to be of avail, a precise diagnosis is, of course, important for prognostic and genetic reasons.

The shape as well as the length of the bones must be assessed, because rickets is a potent inhibitor of skeletal growth. Vitamin D deficiency is rare in the native but not in the immigrant population and responds promptly to supplements. Rickets secondary to renal disease,

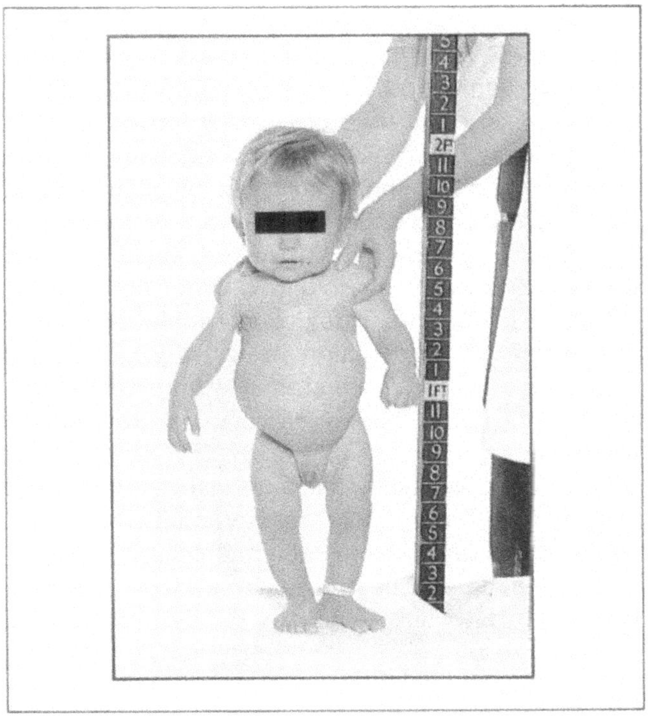

Figure 1.16. *A two-year-old child with short stature due to congenital spondyloepiphysial dysplasia. Note the normal skull, short trunk and normal limbs.*

malabsorption and familial metabolic disorders is also amenable to treatment.

Systemic Disorders

A systematic clinical search for underlying disease of any system must be made in every child with unexplained growth failure. Fortunately, relatively few conditions regularly present in this way without in addition causing reasonably obvious symptoms or signs to draw attention to their presence. Thus there is likely to be little doubt about the underlying problem in children with sufficiently severe heart or lung disease to cause serious growth failure. Renal disease, in contrast, may be silent until a remarkably late stage, but the most difficult disease to exclude and to differentiate from other causes of growth failure is coeliac disease. Symptoms, signs and abnormalities on screening tests for malabsorption may all be absent and so jejunal biopsy must be considered among the most important investigations for obscure growth failure. Other gastrointestinal problems, notably Crohn's disease, may also cause difficulty.

Endocrine Disorders

Although relatively unusual, these are important because they are treatable. Hypothyroidism and hypopituitarism are the two most important causes of endocrine growth failure and these must always be considered in children with an inadequate growth velocity.

Osteogenesis, and therefore growth, provides a sensitive bioassay for adequate levels of circulating thyroid hormones in childhood; retardation of bone age and growth are therefore the cardinal clinical features of hypothyroidism (Figure 1.17). Indeed, these are often the only features; hypothyroid children maintain remarkably good school progress (possibly because of suppression of their natural overactivity!), and they usually lack the whole catechism of symptoms and signs which characterize adult myxoedema. The growth curve of severe hypothyroidism is extremely characteristic showing rapid fall away from a normal growth channel and virtual cessation of bone maturation when hypothyroidism occurs. The hypothyroid child is often expected to be fat but in fact shows an excess of muscle rather than fat which, especially in boys, can cause a misleadingly fit and athletic appearance. The most frequent cause of hypothyroidism in childhood is autoimmune disease, but thyroid dysgenesis, thyroxine biosynthetic defects and other problems may present after the neonatal period. The diagnosis is confirmed by demonstrating a low serum thyroxine and a high, usually very high, serum TSH. A TRH stimulation test and other investigations may be needed in cases of doubt. Replacement treatment, the first and most satisfactory of all endocrine replacements, is extremely simple. Thyroxine given in a dose of approximately 5 μg/kg/day restores complete clinical and biochemical normality. Catch-up growth is remarkable, frequently carrying the child back very rapidly to his genetically appointed growth channel (Figure 1.18).

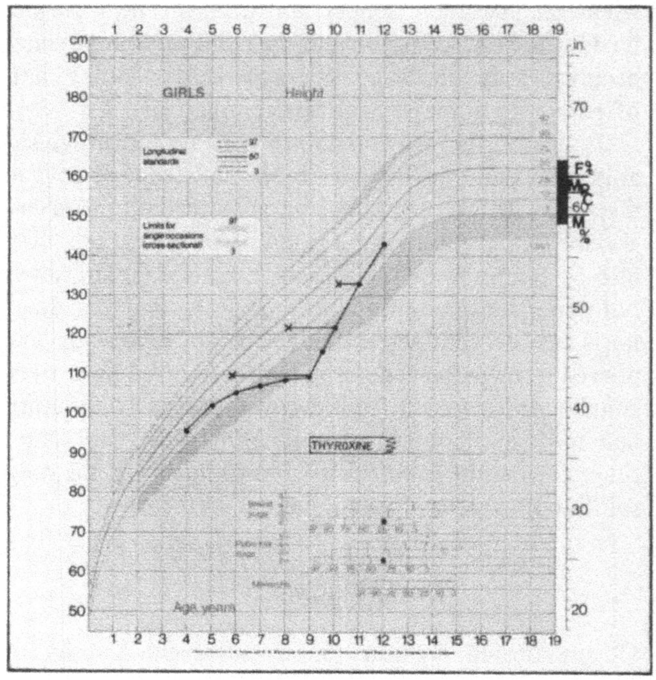

Figure 1.18. *The growth chart of a child with treated hypothyroidism.*

Figure 1.17. *One of these 16-year-old twins proved to be hypothyroid. Note her extreme growth retardation, rounded face and build and delayed development.*

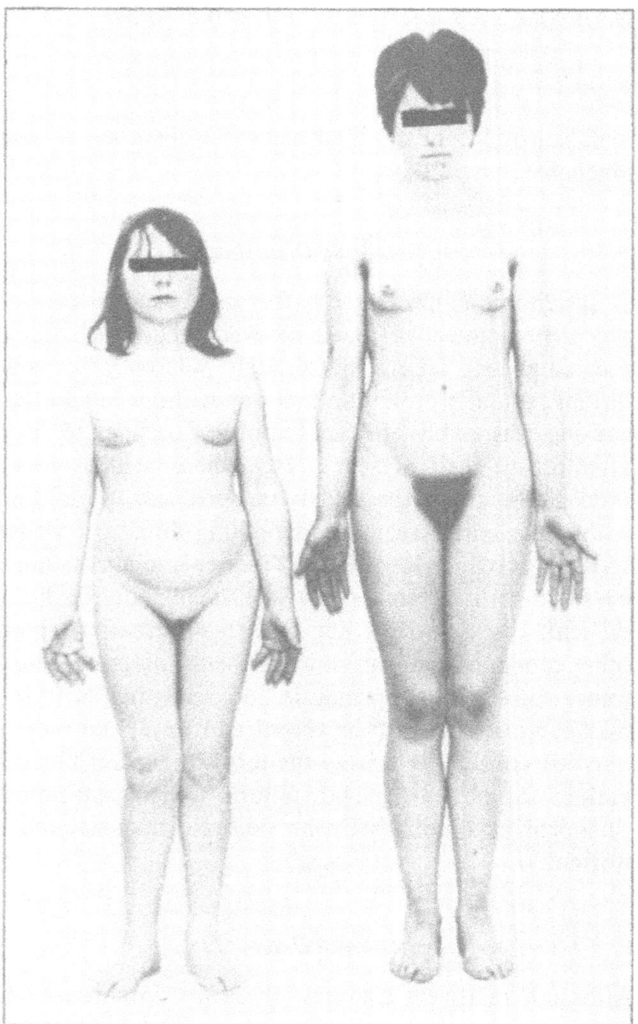

Children with growth hormone deficiency show a wide spectrum of growth retardation which is related to the severity of the endocrine defect. This may be idiopathic or secondary to hypothalamic or pituitary lesions, and it may be isolated or associated with deficiency of other pituitary trophic hormones such as gonadotrophins, ACTH and TSH. Growth hormone deficient children show a low growth velocity and considerable retardation of bone age. They are proportionate and tend to be plump, with a characteristic fat distribution around the trunk, and a lack of muscle tissue. Boys outnumber girls and they often have small genitalia (Figure 1.19). The first impression such children give is often of a fit alert child many years younger than the chronological age. The differential diagnosis from other causes of growth failure can be very difficult, especially in the less severe degrees of growth hormone deficiency, and includes careful assessment of growth velocity, and dynamic testing of pituitary function with insulin-induced hypoglycaemia and other investigations. These are best undertaken by a specialized growth centre, through which supplies of growth hormone can be obtained. The diagnosis should be established as early as possible because prolonged treatment with regular injections of growth hormone is necessary for an acceptable height to be achieved (Figure 1.20).

Treatment with steroids is a potent exogenous cause of endocrine growth failure which merits mention in any discussion of growth problems. The dangers of steroid therapy are now widely appreciated and relatively few children are maintained on high doses for long periods. When this is necessary, growth suppression can be reduced to a minimum by using the smallest effective dose in an alternate day regime, which allows partial recovery of the adrenal axis between doses.

Tall Stature

Tallness is much less frequently a problem than smallness because height is generally considered desirable and relatively few diseases cause excessive growth. The main causes neatly complement those of small stature and are summarized in Table 1.5.

Figure 1.19. *A 15-year-old boy with isolated growth hormone deficiency. Note the proportionate short stature, youthful appearance, fatty trunk, delayed development and small genitalia.*

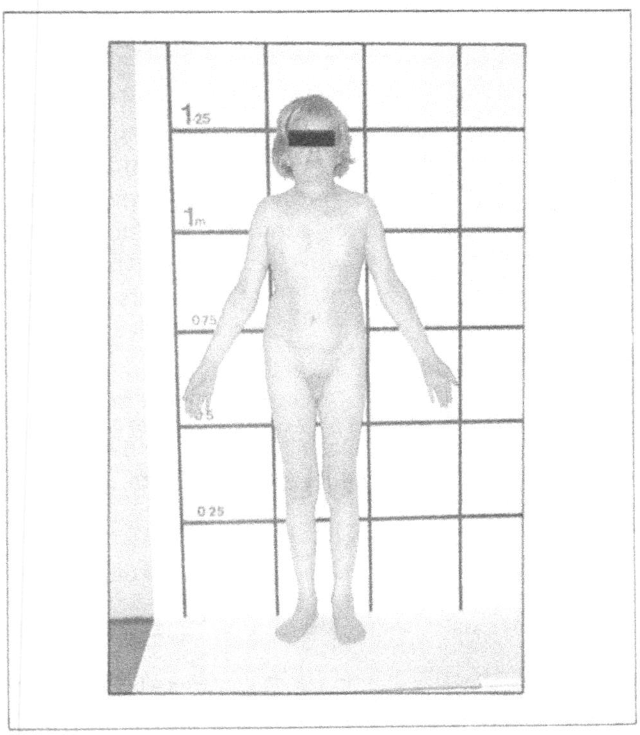

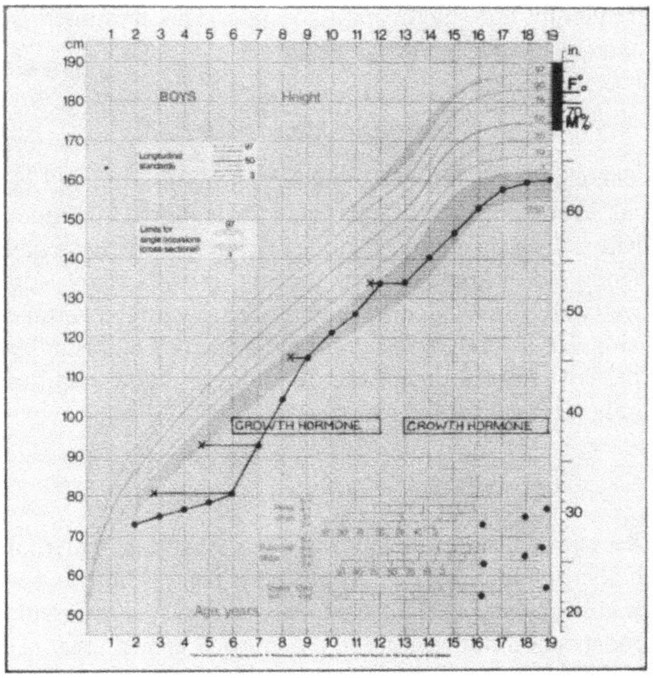

Figure 1.20. *The growth chart of a child with treated growth hormone deficiency.*

Genetic Tall Stature

Tall parents beget tall children; if the parents have found their height an embarrassment or a handicap they will seek advice on limiting their children's growth. The children, who are the beneficiaries of the secular change to increased stature which has occurred in each generation since records have been kept, are often much less disturbed by the prospect of matching their parent's height. Most adolescents, however, will specify a height they would not care to exceed; for boys this is usually 6 ft 4 in or 6 ft 5 in and for girls 5 ft 10 in or 5 ft 11 in. The clinical approach to the problem is identical to that of short stature and, if organic disease can be excluded, a height prediction should be calculated. If this indicates that the child is likely to reach an unacceptable height, growth potential can be limited by acceleration of puberty with exogenous gonadal hormones in high dosage. The administration of oestrogen to girls and testosterone to boys seems, on present evidence, to be safe and reasonably effective. It must, however, be started in early puberty and unfortunately advice is

Table 1.5. Causes of tall stature.

Genetic tall stature
Advanced maturation
Prenatal growth acceleration
Chromosome anomalies
Overnutrition
Skeletal disorders
Endocrine disorders

frequently not sought until too late. This treatment is best supervised by a growth centre.

Advanced Maturation

The child with idiopathic advanced maturation will be tall in comparison with his peers throughout childhood, will enter puberty early and accelerate yet further away from his friends, before ceasing growth early and watching them catch up and, in many cases, overtake him. He is likely to have a family history of a similar pattern of development and, if advice is sought, requires only explanation and reassurance.

Prenatal Growth Acceleration

Recognized causes include large maternal size, maternal diabetes and some dysmorphic syndromes, but, as for small-for-dates infants, frequently no cause is apparent. Most such infants settle into a normal growth channel within several months of birth.

Chromosomal Abnormalities

Two sex chromosome abnormalities predispose to tall stature: Klinefelter's, in which the genetic constitution is XXY and there is testicular dysgenesis with variable hypogonadism and gynaecomastia, and the XYY syndrome, in which tall stature may be associated with personality disorder.

Overnutrition

Overnutrition does cause a slight increase in growth rate with a proportionate advance in the bone age; growth potential is therefore unchanged. In assessing fat children a useful clinical 'rule' states that a tall fat child is normal but a short fat child may well have some underlying disorder.

Skeletal Disorders

These include Marfan's syndrome (Figure 1.21) and other rare disorders in which the habitus is similarly elongated, especially in the extremities.

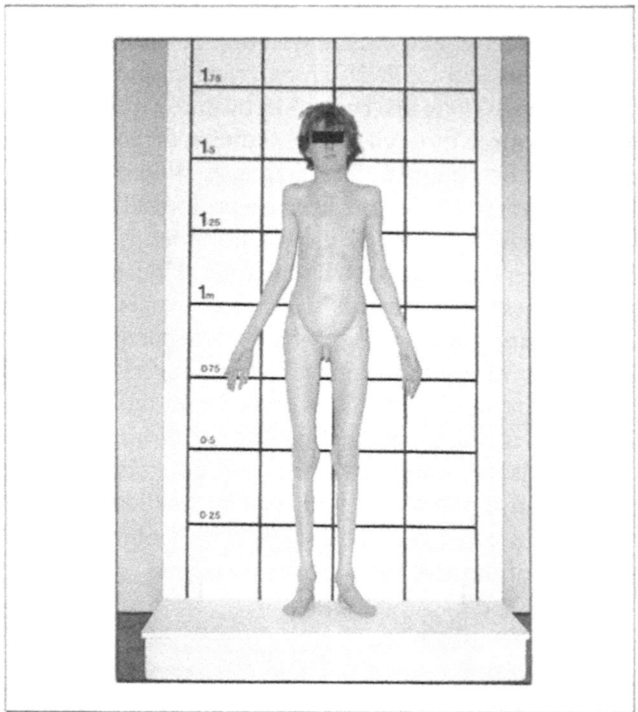

Figure 1.21. *A 12-year-old boy with Marfan's syndrome. Note the tall stature, thin build, long limbs and arachnodactyly.*

Endocrine Disorders

Pituitary gigantism, in which excessive production of growth hormone before puberty causes increased growth without disproportionate acceleration of skeletal development, is fortunately extremely rare. Much more frequent a problem is accelerated growth in childhood due to precocious secretion of gonadal steroids in true precocious puberty, or abnormal secretion of adrenal androgens due to congenital adrenal hyperplasia or a tumour. In these conditions osseous maturation progresses disproportionately fast so that the period of accelerated growth is ended by early fusion of the epiphyses and the final height is short. Prompt diagnosis and treatment is essential for these endocrine disorders and they must be investigated without delay.

Conclusion

The assessment of growth problems thus offers an interesting and clinically rewarding exercise in developmental biology and pathology. Many disorders that present in this way are amenable to treatment, and informed discussion and reassurance is helpful for those that are not. Children with such problems are sufficiently common for general practitioners with an interest in the medicine of childhood to acquire considerable expertise in their management.

Reference

Lacey, K. A., Parkin, J. M., *Arch. Dis. Childh.*, 1974, **49**, 417.

Further Reading

Buckler, J. M. H., *A Reference Manual of Growth and Development*, Blackwell, Oxford, 1979.

Smith, D. W., *Growth and its Disorders*, W. B. Saunders, Philadelphia, 1977.

Tanner, J. M., Physical growth and development, in *Textbook of Paediatrics*, J. O. Forfar and G. C. Arneil (Eds), Churchill Livingstone, Edinburgh, 1978.

2. Immunization

NO topic has provoked more discussion in the last few years than the advantages and dangers of prophylactic immunization in childhood. It is unfortunate that the anxiety that this has generated among the general public has resulted in fewer children being immunized, since elimination on an international scale of diseases such as smallpox, poliomyelitis, diphtheria (Figure 2.1) and yellow fever must rank among the greatest triumphs of medicine. Gillray's comment on the public attitude to Jenner and his vaccine (Figure 2.2) has lost none of its force.

Bacterial Immunization

Diphtheria and Tetanus Immunization

Immunization against these diseases is dependent upon antibodies, produced against toxoids, which cross-react with the bacterial toxins. The toxoids are produced by growing selected strains of *Corynebacterium diphtheriae* (Park-Williams strain) and *Clostridium tetani* (Mueller strain) in liquid media, removing the bacteria and then neutralizing the toxins with formalin in a way which leaves them antigenically intact. To enhance immunogenicity these two toxoids are usually administered adsorbed onto an aluminium salt.

Tetanus immunization was introduced in 1939 and diphtheria immunization in 1942, and the efficacy of these two vaccines has never been in doubt. For tetanus the major benefit was seen during the 1939 to 1945 war, and use of the vaccine allowed injuries, which in the 1914 to 1918 war required amputation to prevent tetanus, to be managed conservatively. The incidence of fatal cases of tetanus in England and Wales during peace-time has also fallen from 81 in 1951 to 0 in 1979. For diphtheria the figures are even more impressive and are shown in Table 2.1. Recent evidence has shown that the antibody titres are well maintained after immunization in infancy and a booster at school entry (Bainton et al. 1979).

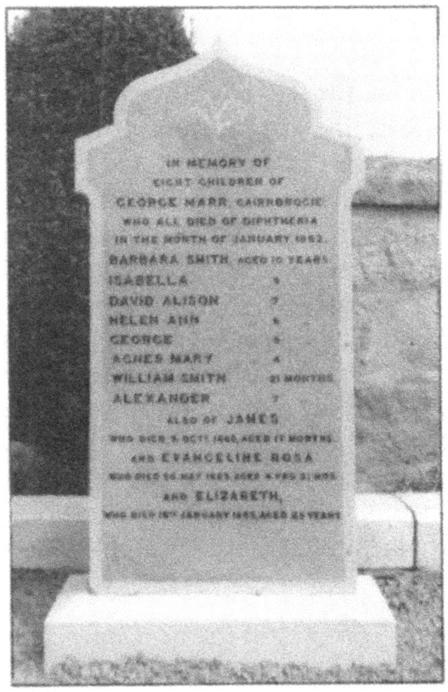

Figure 2.1. *A sad memorial to the previous ravages of diphtheria.*

Pertussis Immunization

In the area of immunization the most heated controversy surrounds pertussis immunization. The chief reason for this is doubt whether the risk of side-effects from the vaccine is greater than the benefits which accrue from its use, particularly as many immunization schedules start after the age at which whooping cough is most serious for infants.

The whole subject was fully discussed in a DHSS publication (DHSS 1977), from which most of the following evidence is derived. (A more recent American review is that of Koplan et al. 1979.) The main facts may be summarized as follows.

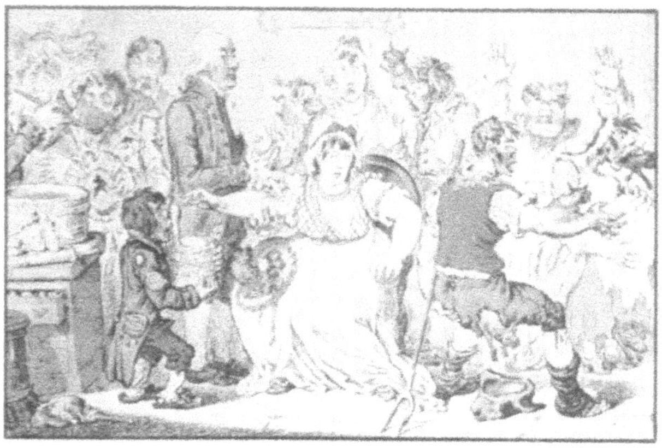

Figure 2.2. *James Gillray's caricature of Edward Jenner and the victims of his vaccine.*

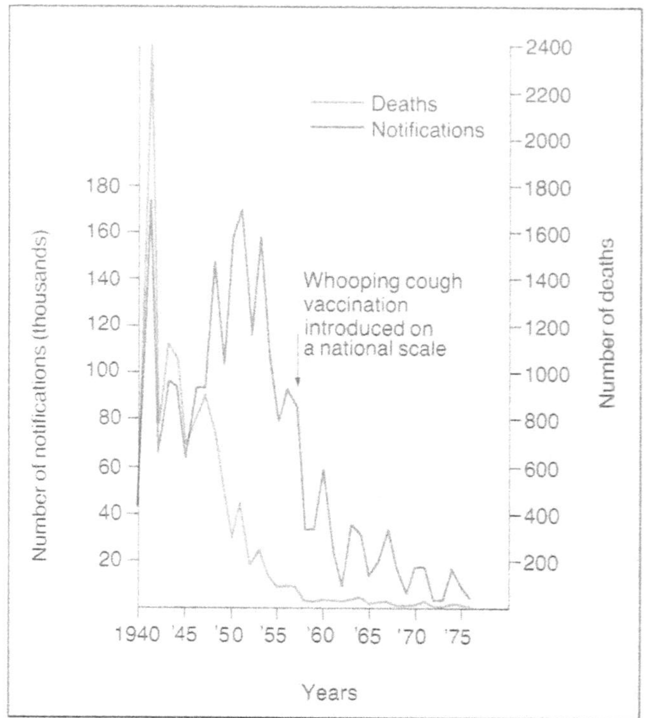

Figure 2.3. *Notifications and deaths from whooping cough in England and Wales, 1940-1976.*

Incidence of Pertussis

Figure 2.3 shows the fall in notifications and fatal cases of pertussis over the last 35 years. It has been pointed out that the decline in incidence and mortality began before the introduction of the vaccine, and it has also been suggested that the continued decline may merely represent further secular improvements in child health and the medical care of affected infants. However, the data from the UK and other sources suggest that the rate of decline accelerated with the introduction of the vaccine. A compelling piece of evidence for the benefits of the vaccine is that since 1978, with the fall in the vaccine acceptance rate, there have been major epidemics of pertussis, with 60,000 notifications that year and approximately 30,000 in 1979 and 1980.

Efficacy of the Vaccine

Some of the early batches of vaccine induced a poor degree of immunity but the currently used vaccine is highly effective.

Table 2.1. Incidence and mortality from diphtheria in England and Wales (from Dudgeon 1976, with permission).

Year	Notifications	Deaths
1940	46,281	2480
	Immunization introduced	
1945	18,596	722
1950	962	49
1960	49	5
1970	22	3
1974	3	0

Timing of Immunization

Severe whooping cough is generally restricted to infants less than six months of age but it is hoped that maintenance of a high level of 'herd immunity' will prevent development of a reservoir of infection in older people from which infants can become infected. The justification for this view is apparent with epidemics occurring now that the level of immunity in the general population has fallen. However, it is no longer thought necessary to withhold immunization until six months, and babies should be immunized from three months of age.

Complications

1. Screaming, irritability and fever after immunization. These symptoms were common with some of the older vaccines but in a continuing study (DHSS 1977) less than one in 1,000 doses of triple vaccine (diphtheria, pertussis and tetanus; DPT) has been followed by this type of reaction, and less than one in 10,000 children has had a fit at this time. Fits in infancy are common (27.2 per 1,000) and it is uncertain whether this incidence is greater than that which would have been expected.

2. Infantile spasms and hypsarrhythmia. Some instances of this neurological syndrome were ascribed specifically to the pertussis component of the triple vaccine. Since the condition frequently results in permanent severe brain damage, it is the one that has engendered most anxiety. Several recent studies (e.g. Melchior 1977), however, have indicated that if infantile spasms are going to develop they do so at the age at which pertussis immunization is usually given in the UK and that changing the time at which pertussis vaccine is administered has no effect upon the incidence, or the age of occurrence of this syndrome.

It is also relevant that infantile spasms can be caused by many other conditions such as phenylketonuria, congenital cytomegalovirus infection and tuberous sclerosis. Some infants whose initial episode of infantile spasms was attributed to pertussis immunization have subsequently been found to have one of these conditions.

Even in the most pessimistic estimates the incidence of this type of complication is less than one per 100,000 doses of vaccine given, and summarizing the evidence, it seems that the association between pertussis vaccine and infantile spasms is unproven.

3. Neurological sequelae in previously brain-damaged children. It has been shown that many of the infants who developed severe neurological sequelae following triple vaccine had clear evidence of pre-existing neurological disease (Kulenkampff et al. 1974). There is no doubt that a family history of fits, previous fits in the infant, the presence of recognized central nervous system malformation or abnormality, or a history of perinatal or postneonatal illness with neurological implication (e.g. birth asphyxia, meningitis, symptomatic hypoglycaemia), are contraindications to the use of pertussis vaccine.

Thus the evidence that pertussis immunization causes significant brain damage or serious sequelae in infants without preceding neurological damage remains unconvincing. We therefore favour the policy that all normal infants should be immunized.

Preparation of the Vaccine

The pertussis vaccine is prepared from cultures of several different strains of *Bordetella pertussis* to provide as broad an antigenic spectrum in the vaccine as possible. Each strain is harvested separately, inactivated in an appropriate way and then incorporated into the vaccine to give approximately 20×10^9 organisms per dose.

Other Bacterial Vaccines

TAB

This vaccine, which is primarily of benefit against typhoid rather than paratyphoid A and B, is not routinely given in the UK. It should be given to any infant more than six months of age who is no longer breast fed and who is travelling outside north-western Europe, North America and the Antipodes. Since most of the malaise and misery that occurs 48 to 72 hours after TAB is due to the paratyphoid component, there is much to be said for using monovalent typhoid vaccine. There are no specific contraindications to either vaccine.

This is a killed bacterial vaccine and administration is commonly followed within 24 to 48 hours by a further one or two days of pyrexia, malaise, myalgia and headache.

Two doses of the vaccine should be given subcutaneously one month apart with booster doses every three to four years. For children under five, 0.1 to 0.3×10^9 organisms are given per injection, which is equivalent to 0.1 to 0.3 ml of the vaccine subcutaneously. For children of five years or over, 0.5 ml should be given on each of two occasions.

Cholera

The cholera vaccine also needs to be given only when travelling to endemic areas. It is a killed bacterial vaccine which should be given subcutaneously in two doses of 0.5 to 1.0 ml (equivalent to 2 to 4×10^9 organisms) one month apart. It is recommended that repeated doses are given every six months for those resident in endemic areas, but it should not be given to children less than 12 months of age. It is a painful injection and has not proved of such great value in controlling outbreaks as was originally believed.

BCG

Bacillus Calmette-Guérin vaccine (BCG) is still routinely given to schoolchildren who are tuberculin negative or show a 1+ positive reaction. Since 1975 the newer 'universal strength' BCG vaccine has been used, 0.1 ml being injected intracutaneously. It should not be given to atopic patients or to those with any primary or acquired immunodeficiency.

In view of the low incidence of tuberculosis in adolescence, and the large number of tuberculin negative schoolchildren, it has been estimated that 1,500 vaccinations are needed to prevent one case of pulmonary tuberculosis. Perhaps, therefore, the routine use of BCG immunization should be reassessed.

However, in areas of the UK where there is a large population of immigrants from the Indian subcontinent, tuberculosis is far from extinct, and still causes considerable morbidity and mortality in early infancy and childhood. In these areas routine neonatal immunization with BCG is carried out.

Clearly, local circumstances must dictate local practices. However, in areas where pulmonary tuberculosis is still a problem, BCG should be used either in the neonatal period or in the school-age population. All health service personnel should be offered immunization.

Pneumococcal Vaccine

A pneumococcal vaccine (Pneumovax) has recently become available which contains capsular polysaccharide antigen from 14 serotypes of pneumococci frequently responsible for serious infections. It is not yet clear how effective the vaccine will prove but it may prevent the majority of pneumococcal disease and should probably be given to children over two years of age who are especially at risk, such as those with nephrotic syndrome, sickle cell disease and asplenia (*Lancet* 1981). 0.5 ml of the vaccine is given subcutaneously and long-lasting immunity is obtained.

Pseudomonas Vaccine

The use of a *Pseudomonas* vaccine has been shown in preliminary trials to benefit burn patients (Jones et al. 1980).

Viral Immunization

Polio Virus

Today it is difficult but salutary to remember the fear which struck a community only 25 years ago when a case or, worse, a series of cases of infantile paralysis was reported. The dangers of death, life in an iron lung, or survival with a withered and useless limb, were well known to all. Yet, currently, the community at large is allowing its level of immunity to fall to an unacceptably low level, and in 1977 the number of confirmed cases of paralytic poliomyelitis was 13, higher than in any of the previous 10 years.

The virtual eradication of this disease has been one of the great successes of modern immunization programmes (Table 2.2). The Salk vaccine, derived from the three major strains of polio virus, was originally used. It is a formalin-inactivated virus grown in monkey kidney cell cultures and its use caused a considerable reduction in the incidence and mortality of poliomyelitis. However, in 1961 the Sabin oral polio vaccine was introduced, a strain attenuated by repeated passage through monkey central nervous system until neurovirulence was lost. It is preferable to the Salk vaccine for several reasons:

1. Oral administration is simpler.

2. Long-lasting immunity from the live vaccine is anticipated.

3. Bowel immunity is induced which leads to elimination of carriers.

4. Shedding of virus from vaccinees acts as a booster for contacts.

However, with Sabin vaccine about 1 in 2 million of those immunized or in contact with a recent vaccinee develops paralytic poliomyelitis, whereas this does not happen with the Salk vaccine. Other complications of immunization are extremely rare with either type of vaccine. It has been suggested that this incidence of paralytic polio following immunization is unacceptable but the current consensus that Sabin vaccine should be used for routine immunization nevertheless remains. There may, however, be a case for the use of Salk vaccine in patients with increased susceptibility to infection due to immunodeficiency or immunosuppression (Nightingale 1977).

One possible difficulty relates to breast feeding. If a mother is breast feeding and is highly immune to polio herself from the administration of the Sabin vaccine within the last two years, she will have a high titre of polio antibody in her breast milk which could attenuate the infant's response to oral polio vaccine. If the infant is only having two or three feeds a day, or the mother is not highly immune, there will be insufficient antibody in the breast milk to affect the response. It is, however, always advisable to give oral polio vaccine as long after the last breast feed as possible.

Table 2.2. Incidence and mortality from paralytic poliomyelitis in England and Wales (from Dudgeon 1976, with permission).

Year	Total cases	Deaths
1950	7760	755
1955	6331	270
	Salk vaccine	
1960	388	46
	Sabin vaccine	
1965	91	3
1970	6	–
1975	3	–

Measles

The dangers of measles also are easily forgotten. In preimmunization years, at least half a million cases occurred per annum, one in 1,000 developed measles encephalitis and some had permanent neurological sequelae. From 1955 to 1965 approximately the same number of children died from measles in epidemic years in the UK as died from asthma. In countries where malnutrition is rife measles is often a fatal disease and mortality rates of five to twelve per cent of affected children have been described.

Where measles vaccine is sufficiently widely accepted to achieve more than 90 per cent immunity in the community, measles epidemics are virtually unknown. In the USA the incidence of the disease has fallen dramatically (Figure 2.4), but in the UK acceptance of the vaccine has been disappointing and there are still approximately 100,000 cases annually (Figure 2.5).

It is now recommended that a single dose of 0.5 ml of the attenuated live measles vaccine of the Schwarz strain is given subcutaneously to all infants over 15 months of age. It should not be routinely combined with immunoglobulin, since this minimizes subsequent immunity. Killed virus vaccine should not be used, since subsequent exposure to wild measles may provoke a severe attack of the disease with features of a type III hypersensitivity reaction. Care should be taken with the vaccine as it rapidly becomes inactivated if not kept in a refrigerator, and many apparent failures of immunization are due to inactive vaccine being administered. Even if the vaccine is properly stored, about 5 per cent of infants fail to develop an immune response to correctly prepared and administered vaccine.

Previous neurological disease or recognized immunodeficiency are contraindications to the use of the vaccine. In infants who have had a single febrile fit, or have an underlying debilitating disease, such as cystic fibrosis or cyanotic congenital heart disease, the live vaccine may be accompanied by 0.5 ml of immune globulin given into the opposite arm. About 10 per cent of children develop a feverish illness and transient morbilliform rash six to twelve days after the injection. Serious neurological sequelae occur with an incidence of approximately one in a million. Immunization with live measles vaccine now is thought to give long lasting immunity, and booster doses are not expected to be necessary.

Figure 2.4. *Notifications of cases of measles and encephalitis from measles in the USA, 1962 to 1976 (from Krugman 1977 with permission).*

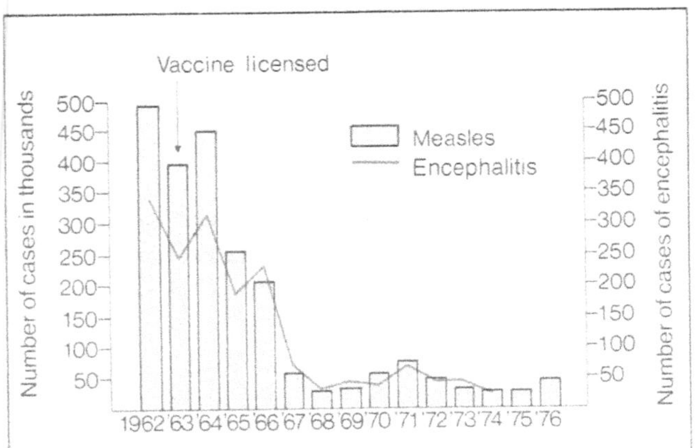

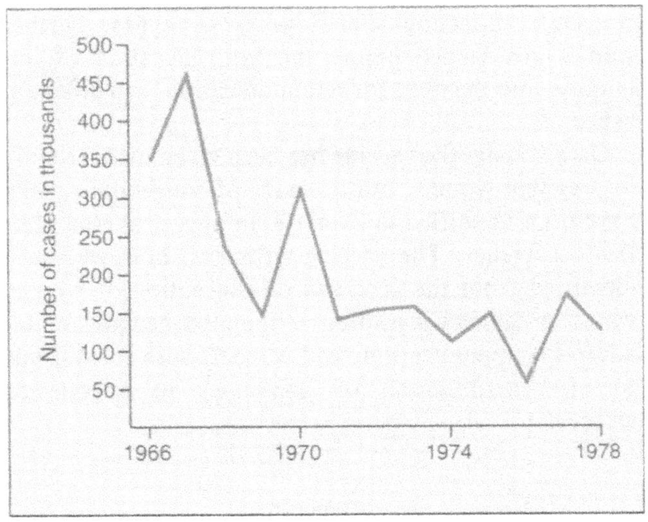

Figure 2.5. *Notifications of cases of measles in England and Wales, 1966-1978.*

Rubella

The purpose of rubella immunization is different since the aim is to ensure that all women are immune during their child-bearing years, so that the danger of congenital rubella is avoided (Krugman 1977). In the USA the vaccine has been given to all children, whereas in the UK only girls between the ages of 11 and 13 years are immunized. In addition, in both countries the vaccine is offered to seronegative women during the puerperium when it should preferably be given in the first 48 hours. Pregnancy is an absolute contraindication to the vaccine because of the possible teratogenic effect on the fetus so women are advised to take contraceptive precautions for one month beforehand, and two months afterwards. A dose of 0.5 ml of the vaccine is given subcutaneously.

In America the effect on the incidence of rubella has been dramatic, but congenital rubella is still seen. In the UK the incidence of congenital rubella continues at a depressingly high level. On average, 67 children with congenital rubella were born in each of the years 1970 to 1973 and no change is yet detectable, and fears have been expressed that a considerable increase may be seen. Satisfactory levels of immunity following immunization have been sustained for at least five years in 95 per cent of vaccinees following the use of either the Cendehill or RA 27/3 strains which are used in this country. These vaccines are associated with fewer side-effects than the HPV 77 strains which were followed by painful persistent arthropathy in as many as 40 per cent of those vaccinated.

The immunity decreases with the passage of time, and reinfection with wild virus can occur, causing an attenuated form of the disease which may very rarely result in congenital infection (Partridge et al. 1981). Further studies are needed before the exact duration of immunity, and the need for reimmunization, can be established.

Occasionally the vaccine has been given inadvertently to pregnant women, but no cases of congenital rubella have been identified in over 100 infants delivered after this occurrence. The vaccine virus has, however, been identified from the products of conception of women whose pregnancy has been terminated because of inadvertent immunization, and it seems wise to continue to offer termination of pregnancy to anyone so affected.

Smallpox

Bangladesh was declared free of smallpox in December 1977 which means that the severe form, variola major, has been eradicated throughout the world. This has been one of the major public health achievements of this century. In 1971 Dick pointed out that many more children suffered severe reactions from smallpox vaccination in the UK than died from the disease, and since that time routine smallpox vaccination has been phased out. It should still be given to health service personnel at high risk of contact (ambulance, casualty and infectious disease unit staff, the latter being especially significant since the recent Birmingham case) and staff of ports and airports. It is contraindicated in those with eczema and care should also be taken if another member of the immediate family has eczema.

Mumps

An effective attenuated mumps virus vaccine is available, but it has not been widely used in the UK although it is extensively used in the USA as a combined vaccine with rubella and measles. It is doubtful whether routine immunization against this virus is justified, however (Dudgeon 1980).

Yellow Fever

A very effective attenuated virus vaccine is available which can be given to children over one year of age, and should be repeated every 10 years in those going to endemic areas.

Influenza

Preparation of vaccines against influenza has been bedevilled by the constantly changing antigenicity of the 'flu viruses. A killed virus vaccine is available which can be used in epidemic years to reduce the incidence of the disease in people at risk, such as NHS employees. It is probably justified to give it to children with chronic lung disease, especially cystic fibrosis. A single subcutaneous dose of the vaccine is recommended.

Other Virus Vaccines

Encouraging preliminary reports on the use of varicella and hepatitis B vaccines have been published, but these are not generally available.

Table 2.3. Suggested immunization schedule.

Age	Vaccine	Interval
3–6 months	DPT and oral polio vaccine (first dose)	
	DPT and oral polio vaccine (second dose)	Preferably after interval of six to eight weeks
	DPT and oral polio vaccine (third dose)	Preferably after interval of four to six months
During the second year of life	Measles vaccine	After interval of not less than three weeks following DPT.
At 5 years of age or school entry	Diphtheria and tetanus and oral polio vaccine	
Between 10 and 13 years of age	BCG vaccine (tuberculin negative children only)	Interval of not less than three weeks between BCG and rubella vaccination.
Girls aged 11 to 13 years	Rubella vaccine	
At 15 to 19 years of age or on leaving school	Polio vaccine (oral or inactivated) and tetanus toxoid.	

Table 2.4. Contraindications to immunization.

Vaccine	Contraindications
All vaccines	—Any acute febrile illness (a common cold or 'snuffles' should not be regarded as a contraindication).
All live vaccines (Measles, oral polio, BCG, rubella, smallpox)	—Pregnancy, particularly early pregnancy, although where there is a significant risk of exposure to serious conditions, such as poliomyelitis, the importance of immunization may outweigh the possible risk to the fetus. —Within three weeks of another live vaccine (but can if absolutely necessary be given on the same day at two different sites). —Immunodeficiency—congenital or acquired. —Malignant disease.
BCG	—Tuberculin positive patients (apart from Heaf Grade 1 reactors). —Eczemas, chronic skin lesions, local sepsis.
Polio	—Gastrointestinal upset. —Allergy to polymyxin, penicillin, streptomycin, or neomycin.
Measles	—Hypersensitivity to egg protein, neomycin or polymyxin. —Children with a history of convulsions, a family history of epilepsy or severe chronic disease should receive simultaneous administration of human normal immunoglobulin with a specific content of measles antibody.
Influenza	—Hypersensitivity to egg protein. —Children under 9 years of age unless serious risks from influenza because of chronic lung or heart disease.
Pertussis	—History of seizures, convulsions or cerebral irritation; history or family history of epilepsy or other diseases of the central nervous system; CNS malformation, neonatal or subsequent brain damage.
Diphtheria	—Severe reaction to a previous dose. —Children more than 10 years of age without a preliminary Shick test to detect the possibility of a serious reaction.
Rubella	—Pregnancy. —Cendevax should not be given to children known to be hypersensitive to rabbits or neomycin. —Almevax should not be given to children known to be hypersensitive to neomycin or polymyxin.
Tetanus	—Booster doses of tetanus should not be given to anyone who is known to have received a booster dose within a year due to possibility of a hypersensitivity reaction.

Immunization Schedules

The immunization schedule recommended in the UK is shown in Table 2.3. The best age at which to start immunization is still debatable. The reasons for the delay until six months of age were to allow maturation of the infant's immune responses and to give time for complete disappearance of transplacentally acquired IgG, which might attenuate the effect of the vaccines. It is now known that three-month-old infants are highly immunocompetent, and that maternal IgG has a half life of about 28 days (although it can be detected for much longer), so these reasons are probably invalid. Reactions to immunization are no worse at three months than at six months, and there are cogent reasons for ensuring that the infant is protected as early as possible, particularly in the third world.

The contraindications to immunization are shown in Table 2.4. It is essential that these are observed, not only because of the dangers to the individual patient, but also because of the bad publicity which results from preventable adverse reactions. This naturally prejudices parents against immunization and so exposes their children unnecessarily to such dangers as crippling by poliomyelitis or severe brain damage and even death from pertussis or measles encephalopathy.

References

Bainton, D., Freeman, M., Magrath, D. I., Sheffield, F. and Smith, J. W. G., *Br. Med. J.*, 1979, **1**, 854.

DHSS, *Whooping Cough Vaccination,* HMSO, London, 1977.

Dick, G., *Br. Med. J.*, 1971, **3**, 163.

Dudgeon, J. A., in *Recent Advances in Paediatrics,* No. 5, D. Hull (Ed.), Churchill Livingstone, Edinburgh, 1976.

Dudgeon, J. A., *Arch. Dis. Childh.*, 1980, **55**, 3.

Jones, R. J., Roe, E. A. and Gupta, J. L., *Lancet,* 1980, **ii**, 1263.

Koplan, J. P., Schoenbaum, S. C., Weinstein, M. C. and Fraser, D. W., *New Engl. J. Med.*, 1979, **301**, 906-911.

Krugman, S., *J. Pediatr.*, 1977, **90**, 1.

Kulenkampff, M., Schwartzman, J. C. and Wilson, J., *Arch. Dis. Childh.*, 1974, **49**, 46.

Lancet (editorial), 1981, **i**, 251.

Melchior, J. C., *Arch. Dis. Childh.*, 1977, **52**, 135.

Nightingale, E. O., *New Engl. J. Med.*, 1977, **297**, 249.

Partridge, J. W., Frewett, T. H. and Whitehead, J. E. M., *Br. Med. J.*, 1981, **2**, 187.

Further Reading

Dick, G., *Immunisation,* Update Books, London, 1978.

Noah, N. D., *Br. J. Hosp. Med.*, 1980, **24**, 533-536.

3. Infant Feeding

FEW, if any, aspects of child care have suffered more buffeting to and fro by the winds of medical fashion than practices in infant feeding. The retrospective knowledge that innumerable 'experts' have advocated innumerable nonsensical practices induces a sense of wariness in us and will, we hope, maintain a due sense of cynicism in our readers! Having stated that, however, we will now risk falling into our own trap by proclaiming that the two major current trends in infant feeding, the return to breast feeding and the production of milk formulae as chemically similar to human milk as possible, seem to be self-evidently and incontrovertibly right.

Comparison between Breast and Bottle Feeding

Psychological and Emotional Aspects

It is difficult to evaluate the differences between breast and bottle feeding from the psychological and emotional points of view, but few would deny that successful breast feeding provides a uniquely intimate and intensely satisfying interaction between mother and baby. There are psychological overtones for the mother, and probably also for the infant, of far greater resonance than the simple 'feeder and fed' relationship. We must, however, acknowledge that unsuccessful breast feeding can provide an intensely unsatisfying and frustrating experience for both mother and baby and the need for appropriate education, guidance and support for mothers is an important aspect of infant feeding which will not be discussed here. Breast feeding propaganda will inevitably generate some feelings of inadequacy in mothers who cannot or do not wish to breast feed.

Chemical Differences

Table 3.1 lists the electrolyte composition of cows' milk, breast milk, an old-fashioned unmodified cows' milk

Table 3.1. Mineral content of milks.

	Cows'	Full Cream Cow and Gate	Cow and Gate Premium	Osterfeed	Milumil	SMA Gold Cap	Breast
Sodium							
mEq/l	25	23	10	8.5	12.5	6.5	6.4
mg/100 ml	55	52	22	19	27	15	15
Potassium							
mEq/l	36	29	15	14.5	21.5	14.3	15
mg/100 ml	140	115	60	57	86	56	60
Calcium							
mg/100 ml	130	105	48	44	71	44	35
Magnesium							
mg/100 ml	13	x	4.5	5.2	7	5.3	13
Phosphate							
mg/100 ml	100	80	31	31	55	33	15

x Data not available

based formula (full cream Cow and Gate) and the four commonly used new formulae (Cow and Gate Premium, SMA Gold Cap, Osterfeed and Milumil). It can be seen that cows' milk and the unmodified milk have much higher sodium, potassium, calcium and phosphate levels than the newer milks and, of course, higher levels than breast milk.

In the neonatal period, cows' milk and unmodified milks induce hyperphosphataemia which may cause neonatal hypocalcaemia and convulsions in as many as one in every 200 babies. Breast feeding, or alternatively the use of a low phosphate milk, virtually eliminates the occurrence of these fits.

The high solute load of cows' milk and unmodified formulae exposes infants to the risk of hypernatraemia, uraemia and hyperosmolarity, which may occur not only when gastroenteritis causes frank dehydration but also when there is marginally increased insensible water loss for any reason. These metabolic derangements may lead to convulsions and brain damage and it is possible that this sequence of events may contribute to some cases of cot death. It may also initiate a vicious circle of thirst and over-feeding: the hyperosmolarity makes the baby thirsty but his cry is interpreted as hunger, and instead of being offered the water he needs, he is given more milk or high solute solid food. This aggravates the problem and the concomitant calorie intake may result in excessive weight gain (Figure 3.1). These dangers were first recognized in infants fed on unmodified cows' milk formulae which had been incorrectly prepared with excess powder. If the milks are prepared correctly and cereals are not added, hyperosmolarity is less likely to occur.

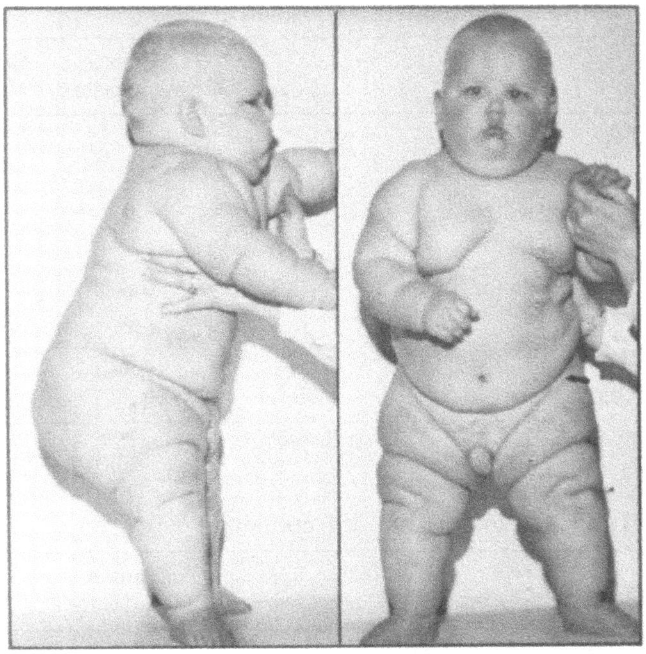

Figure 3.1. *Overfed babies can become very fat.*

Nutritional Differences

Tables 3.2 and 3.3 show nutritional differences between milks. Nutritional superiority of breast milk in comparison with cows' milk is not well documented and little evidence is available that there are long-term benefits to breast fed infants. All the milks give approximately the same number of calories. Cows' milk has a much higher casein to lactalbumin ratio than breast milk, and the higher casein content predisposes to curd formation in the stomach and increases the solute load, once again with the risk of uraemia and hyperosmolarity. The newer milks have a lower protein content and a more appropriate casein to lactalbumin ratio. The amino acid composition of cows' milk protein is different from that of breast milk, but it is not known whether this is important in the long term.

We are similarly ignorant about the importance of the fat content. The relatively similar total fat content shown in Table 3.2 disguises major differences in the fatty acid composition of the different milks. There is much more long-chain saturated fat in cows' milk, which chelates more calcium in the gut and thus prevents its absorption, and the different fatty acid composition in cows' milk derived formulae may possibly predispose to important late nutritional problems including atherosclerosis. Lactose is the carbohydrate in all the milks except Milumil, which contains some glucose polymers—maltidextrins. Recent evidence suggests that if a mother's iron status is adequate the baby will obtain adequate amounts of iron from breast milk (Saarinen and Siimes, 1979) and that breast milk also contains large amounts of water-soluble vitamin D (Lakdawala and Widdowson, 1977).

The Role of Milk in the Prevention of Infection

The most impressive advantages of breast over bottle milk are related to the prevention of infection. These apply particularly to the gut and organisms from it, such as *E. coli,* which not only cause gastroenteritis but, in the neonatal period, can also cause septicaemia, meningitis and renal disease. Breast milk does not, of course, render the gut sterile but keeps the content of pathogenic organisms at an acceptably low level.

One way in which breast milk exerts an anti-infective action is through its effect on colonic pH. Cows' milk, with its high protein and phosphate content, is an effective buffer but breast milk is not, so the stools of the breast fed infant are acidic with a pH of 5 compared with 7 in bottle fed babies. *E. coli* does not thrive in an acid environment, and the stool *E. coli* count is therefore low in breast fed babies. The new formulae, with a

Table 3.2. Nutritional composition of milks.

	Cow	Full Cream Cow and Gate	Cow and Gate Premium	Osterfeed	Milumil	SMA Gold Cap	Breast
Fat (g/100 ml)	3.8	3.1	3.45	3.8	3.1	3.6	4.2
Protein	3.3	3.0	1.8	1.45	1.9	1.5	1.1
Casein	2.7	2.5	0.57	0.56		0.6	0.37
Lactalbumin (g/100 ml)	0.6	0.5	1.23	0.89		0.9	0.73
Lactose	4.7	4.2	6.9	7.0	8.4*	7.2	7.4
Sucrose (g/100 ml)		3.3					
Calories (per 100 ml)	65	68	65	68	68	65	70

*This is a mixture of lactose and maltidextrins

Table 3.3. Vitamin and iron content of milks.

	Cow	Full Cream Cow and Gate	Cow and Gate Premium	Osterfeed	Milumil	SMA Gold Cap	Breast
Vitamin D (μg/100 ml)	0.5	1.0	1.1	1.0	1.0	1.05	0.8[1]
Vitamin A (μg/100 ml)	17–38	100	79	40	61	79	60
Vitamin E (μg/100 ml)	60	x	1000	480	600	950	350
Iron (mg/100 ml)	0.15	0.40	0.65	0.96	0.7	1.27	0.08
Folate (μg/100 ml)	3.7	x	3.5	5.0	10	5.3	5.2

[1] Water soluble vitamin D
x Data not available

lower protein and phosphate content than unmodified cows' milk, have an intermediate action in this respect. Breast milk also contains a glycoprotein known as the 'bifidus factor' which is an essential nutrient for the non-pathogenic lactobacillus species which therefore becomes the predominant organism in the gut, at the expense of *E. coli,* and also produces lactate, further lowering the pH and preventing *E. coli* overgrowth.

Immunoglobulin A

There are also more specific anti-infective factors in breast milk which cannot be added by the baby-milk manufacturers' chemists. The most important of these is immunoglobulin A (IgA). This immunoglobulin, which protects exposed mucosal surfaces, is secreted into breast milk and exerts a protective effect on the gastrointestinal tract in several ways. It agglutinates bacteria in the gut, prevents the adherence of bacteria to the gut wall, which is a necessary step before gastroenteritis can develop, interacts with lactoferrin and may neutralize toxins. In addition, in the presence of complement and lysozyme, which are also found in breast milk, it can cause bacterial cell lysis and, coupled with complement and white cells, can cause bacterial ingestion and destruction. IgA is present in high concentrations in colostrum, and although it is much more dilute in mature breast milk, the volume of milk ingested is so great that the absolute amount the infant receives daily remains high. One of the most remarkable biological features of the IgA system is the fact that the lymphocytes which make the IgA in the breast are derived from the mother's gut. The infant's gastrointestinal tract is therefore protected by the same IgA which protects the mother's, thus giving him protection against the flora to which he will be particularly exposed. Furthermore, the more exposure to enteric pathogens the mother has, the higher the level of IgA in her breast milk.

There is also some IgG in breast milk, the role of which is uncertain, and low levels of IgM. Complement, lysozyme and lactoperoxidase are all present in breast milk and interact with the breast milk immunoglobulins to promote bacterial cell lysis.

Presence of White Blood Cells

Another important anti-infective factor is the presence of white cells in breast milk. Lymphocytes, polymorphs and macrophages are present and carry out the same phagocytic and immunoglobulin-producing functions that they have elsewhere. Polymorphs in particular may

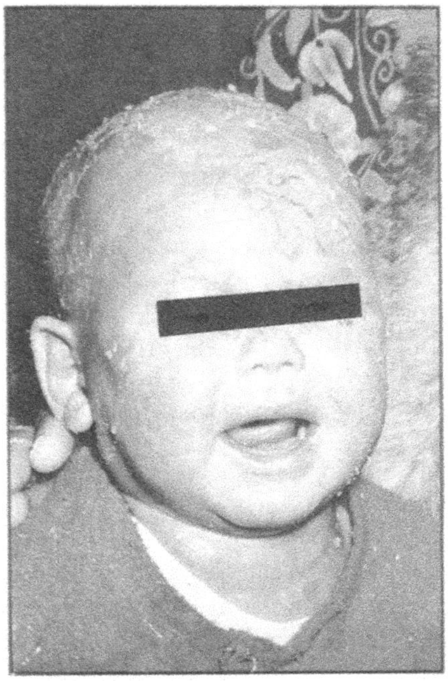

Figure 3.2. *An infant with severe eczema who proved to be allergic to cows' milk.*

be important in removing *E. coli* which have been opsonized by IgA and complement.

Other Anti-infective Factors

Breast milk contains anti-viral agents including antibodies to the common gut pathogen, the rotavirus. Interferon is also present, and recently a specific low molecular weight protein has been identified which inhibits viral multiplication in tissue culture. It is likely that these factors are partly responsible for the decreased incidence of respiratory infection in breast fed babies.

Another interesting component of breast milk is lactoferrin. This is a protein with a high capacity for binding iron in the presence of IgA. This action renders the gut lumen virtually iron free and bacteria, including *E. coli*, deprived of iron, are no longer able to multiply. Similar proteins have been identified which bind folic acid and vitamin B_{12}.

It has always been assumed that one major reason for the benefit of breast feeding in relation to infection lies in the greater cleanliness of its mode of delivery. This is probably no longer true in countries where most families are able to maintain a high standard of cleanliness during the preparation of infant feeds, but it certainly remains important where suitable facilities are not available.

Other Differences

Allergy

Allergy to cows' milk protein is much less likely to develop if the infant has not been exposed to it during the first few months of life. Preliminary studies have also suggested that other manifestations of allergic disease, such as eczema (Figure 3.2), may be minimized by the use in the early months of life of a hypoallergenic diet, which includes avoidance of cows' milk derived proteins (Matthew et al. 1977).

Cost and Convenience

The relative convenience of breast feeding and bottle feeding is an individual matter. Some mothers are uninhibited about breast feeding in public places, but many feel inhibited even in front of members of their family. Since wetnurses are no longer available, breast feeding is one task which cannot be delegated. As far as cost is concerned, although the breast feeding mother does need to ingest extra calories, she can do so in the form of relatively inexpensive foods and there can be little doubt that breast feeding is now cheaper than bottle feeding.

Cot Death

It has been claimed that cot death occurs more commonly in bottle fed than breast fed babies. Recent reappraisal of the evidence, however, suggests that the association is not as strong as was formerly believed.

Disadvantages of Breast Feeding

The few disadvantages of breast feeding must not be forgotten. For the small-for-dates infant at risk from hypoglycaemia, breast feeding may not provide adequate calories during the first 48 to 72 hours of life, and complementary feeds must be given.

Until lactation is well established the breasts may be uncomfortable due to engorgement, the nipples may become cracked and breast abscess remains common.

Drugs the mother is taking will pass into breast milk and can affect the baby. In a few instances this matters, including the passage of lithium, alcohol and some anticoagulants. Sedative and psychotropic drugs also pass into breast milk, but usually in small amounts only, and if the mother is keen to breast feed she should be encouraged to do so while the baby is watched for signs of drowsiness and other side-effects.

The average mother produces 800 to 1,000 ml of breast milk daily (Coward et al. 1979), which provides 170 ml/kg/24 hours for a 5 kg baby. Since some breast fed babies weigh more than this and some mothers produce less milk than the average, it is important to check weight gain regularly.

There is no doubt that some breast fed babies do receive a grossly inadequate intake (Figure 3.3) until complementary or supplementary feeds are introduced and some tolerate such deprivation with remarkable equanimity. Breast fed babies need more frequent feeds and for this reason they need a night feed for longer than those who are bottle fed.

Feeding Problems

We will now briefly consider some of the more common difficulties which beset the apparently straightforward matter of infant feeding.

Volume of Milk and Weight Gain

On average, an infant in the first few months of life requires 170 ml of milk per kg body weight per day ($2\frac{1}{2}$ oz/lb). He should gain about 30 g (1 oz) per day for the first six months of life, slightly less towards the end of this period, and during the second six months of life about 15 to 20 g per day. The most common cause of poor weight gain in infancy is inadequate intake, and the number of feeds offered per 24 hours, the correctness of their preparation, and the volume retained should always be established in bottle fed babies who are not gaining weight adequately. In breast fed babies one or two test weighings will usually prove an adequate guide to the amount of milk produced by the mother. There is no point in excessively frequent weighing of the baby and indeed in breast fed infants it has been shown to inhibit lactation.

Figure 3.3. *A marasmic breast fed African infant.*

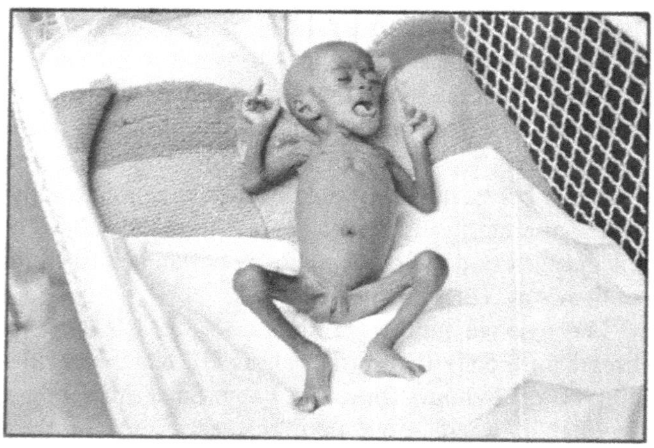

Frequency of Feeds

Bottle fed babies usually settle into a routine of feeding every four hours but it is important to remember, and to inform mothers that most breast fed babies require extra feeds. This lends itself to the development of demand feeding, which ensures that the baby is alert and keen for his feed, has not been crying for a long time so that he has become windy and upset, and has not been roused from deep sleep, when nobody, least of all a newborn baby, feels like tucking into a meal. If a breast fed baby requires frequent feeds, this is not an indication that the mother's lactation is inadequate or that supplementary bottle feeds or solids are needed.

Solids

There is no reason to introduce solids into the baby's diet before three months at the earliest. There is no evidence that solids are needed nutritionally before this age and none that giving the baby solids in the evening helps him to sleep through the night sooner rather than later. With solids there is increased risk of hyperosmolarity. Furthermore, solids and the proteins they contain may predispose to food allergy. In particular, coeliac disease is more likely to develop when the infant is exposed to gluten early in life.

Crying Babies

It must be remembered that babies cry for reasons other than hunger: they may be wet or dirty, they may be cross because they are already social animals and want company, or they may be in pain or unwell. There is no doubt that a tense mother can produce a tense baby and a vicious circle can thus be set up. However, many crying and irritable babies seem simply to have been born that way and are not the result of poor handling. In this situation the mother needs patient support and reassurance. Many such babies are labelled as 'colicky'. These infants scream and draw their legs up especially after the evening feed. The symptoms can be very persistent, and if they are not relieved by antispasmodics, such as Merbentyl (dicyclomine hydrochloride), and the infant is gaining weight well, all that can be done is to support the mother until the infant grows out of the problem at three to four months of age. A crying baby may indeed be hungry, and an experienced mother rapidly learns to recognize the hunger cry of her own infant. However, thirst is also an important cause of crying and especially in hot weather, with fever, or if the baby is on solids or an unmodified milk preparation, a drink of water should be offered as an alternative to a further bottle. Swopping from one milk to another is of no value in the treatment of crying, irritable infants.

Wind

When a mother says her baby is 'windy', she usually means that it seems to have colic and abdominal pain, often in association with much rumbling and the passage of an excessive quantity of gas from one end or the other. Babies swallow air if they cry a lot before they are fed. If bottle fed they may suck in a lot of air with the milk as the bottle empties. If the teat has too small a hole they may suck so hard that they draw air in round it, and if it has too large a hole they may gulp down milk and air too rapidly. This may also occur if there is poor apposition of the lips to the mother's areola during breast feeding. Prolonged winding of the baby, however, merely leads to maternal and infant exhaustion. If the infant does not burp within minutes of being winded it is unlikely that much wind will be produced since it will have passed the pylorus.

Slow Feeders

Some babies are just slow. In others the problem may be due to the mother interrupting the feed by taking the bottle out of the baby's mouth too often to try to wind him. If there is too small a hole in the teat, the baby has to work for a long time to get an adequate volume of milk. Slow feeding can be a sign that the baby is ill. It may also result from an obstructed nostril, due either to upper respiratory tract infection or rarely to congenital malformation, and it may be an indication that the child has poor neurological co-ordination.

Vomiting

The sudden onset of vomiting usually indicates an acute illness, such as an infection in the respiratory, gastrointestinal or urinary tract. After the neonatal period it only rarely indicates intestinal obstruction but obstruction should be considered if the vomiting is bilious or faeculant, or if there is coexistent abdominal distention or constipation. Intussusception must be especially kept in mind.

When vomiting is persistent, it is important to ascertain whether the infant is gaining weight normally (Figure 3.4). If it is, then the most likely diagnosis is simple regurgitation, which will resolve spontaneously and is relieved by avoiding over-feeding and by thickening the milk feeds with a preparation such as Carobel. If the infant is not gaining weight well, the many causes of failure to thrive should be considered (see chapter 1).

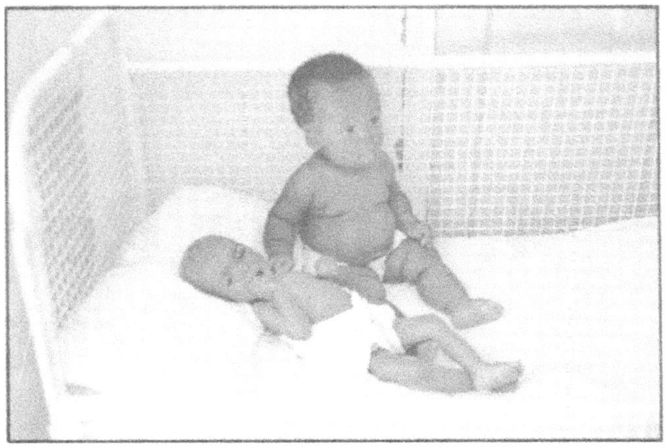

Figure 3.4. *Two eight-month-old breast fed African infants showing a contrast in nutritional states.*

Persisting Feeding Difficulties

There are some feeding problems which seem to be insoluble; in spite of all efforts the infant continues to scream, vomit, feed badly or gain weight poorly. The extreme maternal and family stress that can arise in this situation makes it all too easy to understand how such infants may come to be battered. It is certainly a fully justified use of a hospital bed to admit such an infant for a short period. He can then be given an appropriate caloric intake and be fed by dispassionate nurses. Under the supervision of sympathetic and experienced nursing staff most feeding problems are soon resolved. If the infant still does not gain weight then appropriate further investigation will be needed.

References

Coward, W. A., Sawyer, M. B., Whitehead, R. G., Prentice, A. M. and Evans, J., *Lancet,* 1979, **ii**, 13.

Lakdawala, D. R. and Widdowson, E. M., *Lancet,* 1977, **i**, 167.

Matthew, D. J., Taylor, B., Norman, A. P., Turner, M. W. and Soothill, J. F., *Lancet,* 1977, **i**, 321.

Saarinen, U-M. and Siimes, M. A., *Pediatr. Res.,* 1979, **13**, 143.

Further Reading

DHSS, *Present Day Practice in Infant Feeding,* HMSO, London, 1974.

Gunther, M., *Infant Feeding,* Methuen, London, 1970.

4. Upper Respiratory Tract Problems

UPPER respiratory tract problems are common throughout childhood; indeed, this is by far the most frequent site of infection at all ages, most children suffering several upper respiratory tract infections annually. Much of this illness is trivial but it may occasionally be life-threatening. The pattern of disease is, as usual in paediatrics, largely determined by the age of the child. For example, infants are less susceptible to group A beta-haemolytic streptococci than are their older siblings, but are much more likely to develop serious illness with the respiratory syncytial virus or the para-influenza virus. Some of the factors which determine the pattern of disease are apparent, such as changing anatomical relationships and the stage of development of the lymphoid system, but most remain as obscure as the complex interaction of genetic, environmental and immune mechanisms which determine individual susceptibility to infection.

We will consider some of the commoner and more important upper respiratory tract problems, somewhat arbitrarily divided into those primarily affecting the nose, the ear and the throat.

Nasal Problems

'Colds'

A wide variety of viruses, including the rhino, respiratory syncytial, para-influenza and influenza viruses, can cause the upper respiratory tract infection syndrome of acute nasopharyngitis, coryza or the common cold. The peak incidence is around the age of five years but the symptoms tend to be more severe in younger infants. The onset of fever, which may rise to as high as 40°C, is followed by a serous nasal discharge which subsequently becomes purulent without bacterial super-infection. There is generalized inflammation of the upper respiratory tract with hyperaemia and oedema of the mucosa. The swelling and secretions cause nasal obstruction which renders the infant, who requires a patent nasal airway for feeding, unable to maintain sustained sucking from breast or bottle. His fluid intake therefore falls and, combined with the effects of fever and sometimes vomiting, this is likely to lead to dehydration. It is in just such circumstances as these that infants fed on unmodified milk formulae or solids can develop serious hypernatraemia and hyperosmolarity and are prone to all the complications of hypernatraemic dehydration, from brain damage to cot death.

Since there is generalized inflammation of the upper respiratory tract mucosa, the ear drums are often congested. This does not indicate bacterial infection and usually resolves rapidly. True otitis media is, however, the commonest complication of the cold and is seen most frequently in infants. It usually presents after the acute phase of the cold is over.

Treatment

There is no specific therapy for this viral illness so treatment can only be symptomatic. Antibiotics do not affect the course of the illness or reduce the incidence of bacterial complications but are nevertheless grossly over-used (Stott 1979). An adequate fluid intake with allowance for losses must be maintained. The fever and generalized aching usually respond to small doses of aspirin or paracetamol. Relief of the nasal obstruction is necessary to allow infants to feed and sleep. It is best achieved by local instillation of vasoconstricting drops, such as 0.5 per cent ephedrine, one or two drops into each nostril 15 minutes before feeds and at bedtime. When instilling the drops, it is important to position the child on his back with neck extended to ensure that the drops reach the right place and it may be necessary to add a further drop five minutes later to clear the whole nasal airway. This treatment should not be continued for more than two or three days.

In older children the symptoms are less severe and resemble those which occur in adults. Parents often expect children to recover very rapidly (Stott 1979) so it is worth emphasizing that the acute phase may last from four to ten days. In susceptible children such virus infections frequently trigger wheeziness and lower respiratory tract complications. The management of these will be considered in chapters 5 and 6.

Chronic Rhinitis

Atopic children often have seasonal rhinitis with a profuse watery discharge, paroxysms of sneezing and red, watery eyes—symptoms which are clearly related to the prevailing pollen count and are recognized by all as hay fever. However, the perennial incidence of similar symptoms is often ascribed by parents to 'continuous colds, doctor'. Such children are habitual mouth breathers and sniffers and often show the characteristic transverse crease across the nose which results from rubbing the tip upwards. The nasal mucosa, best seen through a large auroscope, has a pale, boggy, swollen appearance and occasionally polyps may be present. The secretions show a high eosinophil count. Some children are allergic to the house dust mite or to animal danders in which case avoidance measures and desensitization may be helpful but, more commonly, specific allergens cannot be identified and treatment must be symptomatic. Antihistamines are often effective but have a sedative effect. This unwanted side-effect often lessens with continued use but it is obviously important that the treatment should not be more troublesome than the disease. Children often tolerate the symptoms well and it is undesirable to reduce their alertness simply to make them socially more acceptable! Local treatment by instillation of cromoglycate or steroid drops or sprays into the nose and/or eyes can also be effective but only a minority of children voluntarily persist with such treatment.

Chronic rhinitis may also be due to a foreign body, infected adenoids, chronic sinusitis or anatomical blockage due to a deviated septum or unilateral choanal atresia.

Nose Bleeds

Nose bleeds are rare in infancy but common throughout the rest of childhood. The site of bleeding is usually the mucosa of the anterior septum, which has a rich anastomotic blood supply. The commonest cause is trauma, including picking of the nose. The incidence of bleeding is increased in children with rhinitis. Bleeding may occasionally indicate the presence of a tumour or polyp, a bleeding disorder or hypertension. Compression of the nose with cold packs while sitting upright and breathing through the mouth usually helps stop the bleeding but internal packing is sometimes necessary. Cautery of the vessels on the mucosa may relieve the tendency. Swallowed blood may cause confusion when it is vomited or passed in the stools.

Choanal Atresia

This rare congenital malformation must be recognized without delay because newborn infants are obligatory nose breathers and so bilateral complete atresia may be rapidly fatal. An affected infant makes violent inspiratory efforts but fails to achieve any air entry unless his mouth is open. The diagnosis is confirmed if it proves impossible to pass a catheter or probe into the nasopharynx. In an emergency an airway can be established simply by propping the jaws open and most infants soon learn to breathe through their mouths. The atresia is usually bony so surgery is necessary to establish a nasal airway.

Ear Problems

Acute Otitis Media

Bacterial pathogens play the major role in this infection. About half of the cases are due to the *Pneumococcus* and one quarter to *Haemophilus influenzae*, which is more frequent in the younger age-groups. The remaining cases are due to viral infections, staphylococci, streptococci or *Mycoplasma*. The infection enters the middle ear cleft via the eustachian tube and infants are particularly susceptible, probably because they spend much time lying supine and their eustachian tubes are relatively short, horizontal and easily obstructed at the entrance. Children with cleft palate or palatal dysfunction are particularly prone to otitis media.

Otitis media is predominantly an infection of the winter months and often follows another infection such as a cold, tonsillitis or measles. The main symptoms are fever and pain, the latter localized to the ear in older children but simply causing misery and irritability in infants who, as in other upper respiratory tract infections, may also have a misleading amount of vomiting and diarrhoea. At first, the tympanic membrane is acutely inflamed and then, as purulent secretions accumulate behind it, bulges into the meatus and loses its landmarks.

Management

The management of acute suppurative otitis media has been the subject of many controlled trials. These have shown that antibacterial therapy is definitely indicated but that there is little to choose between penicillin, ampicillin, sulphonamides or co-trimoxazole given either parenterally or orally. In acute illness, and especially in the presence of vomiting, it seems wise to give an initial injection of parenteral penicillin G followed by oral penicillin for at least 10 days. Ampicillin or co-trimoxazole are logical first-line drugs in infants, who are more likely to harbour *Haemophilus*, but are not demonstrably superior to penicillin. Reliable bacteriological proof that a certain pathogen is involved requires aspiration of the middle ear cavity, which is clearly not a practical proposition in the majority of cases. It is, therefore, important to review the child three or four days into the illness and to change the antibiotic if necessary.

Another logical measure is to prescribe a nasal decongestant, given either orally or by local instillation, in the hope that it will promote drainage of the middle ear cleft, but the value of this is unproven. Nevertheless, we generally recommend nasal drops to be given for the first few days of the illness. Acceptable relief of the pain can usually be achieved with simple analgesics. With early diagnosis and effective antibiotic therapy, myringotomy is seldom needed but provides dramatic relief of the pain and should certainly be considered in unresolved otitis. Prophylactic treatment with a sulphonamide or penicillin through the winter months may sometimes be helpful in children with recurrent otitis media.

Complications

The complications of otitis media which were familiar to all doctors are now seldom seen. The disease may resolve by perforation of the ear drum but, if it is vigorously treated, progression to chronic suppurative otitis media can generally be prevented. However, mastoiditis (Figure 4.1) and the intracranial complications, such as thrombophlebitis, meningitis and abscess formation, still occur. Although it is not clear just how great is the contribution of unresolved acute otitis media to the problem of serous otitis, this is probably the most frequent complication.

Serous Otitis Media

Otherwise known as secretory otitis or glue ear, this is by far the most common cause of hearing loss in childhood, with a peak incidence from five to eight years of age. The accumulation of serous fluid in the middle ear seems to occur largely as a physical phenomenon secondary to blockage of the eustachian tube but several other factors, such as allergy, viral infections and unresolved bacterial otitis are likely to play a part. The condition is usually bilateral and deafness is the only important symptom. Audiography shows that the deafness is conductive and variable in extent; there is generally about a 30 to 50 decibel loss across the whole frequency range. The appearance of the tympanic membrane is variable and often difficult to interpret, with dullness, bulging or retraction, injected vessels, fluid levels or even an essentially normal appearance.

Many cases resolve spontaneously and, once again, decongestants are the logical treatment although they are of unproven value. Removal of the adenoids or treatment of allergy or chronic infection may sometimes be helpful but, in established cases, myringotomy and aspiration of the secretions are required. This usually restores hearing rapidly (Figure 4.2). In recurrent or persistent cases it is current practice to insert small plastic tubes (grommets) in the tympanic membranes to allow equalization of pressure. These usually remain in place for some months before they are spontaneously extruded. Their proposed function is to prevent re-accumulation of fluid and progressive fibrosis of the middle ear structures with permanent loss of hearing.

Figure 4.1. *This infant presented with a large post-auricular swelling which proved, in spite of the age of the patient and the site of the swelling, to have originated in the mastoid.*

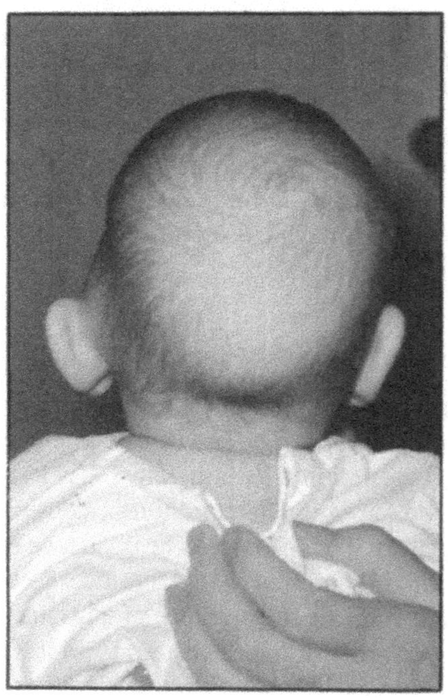

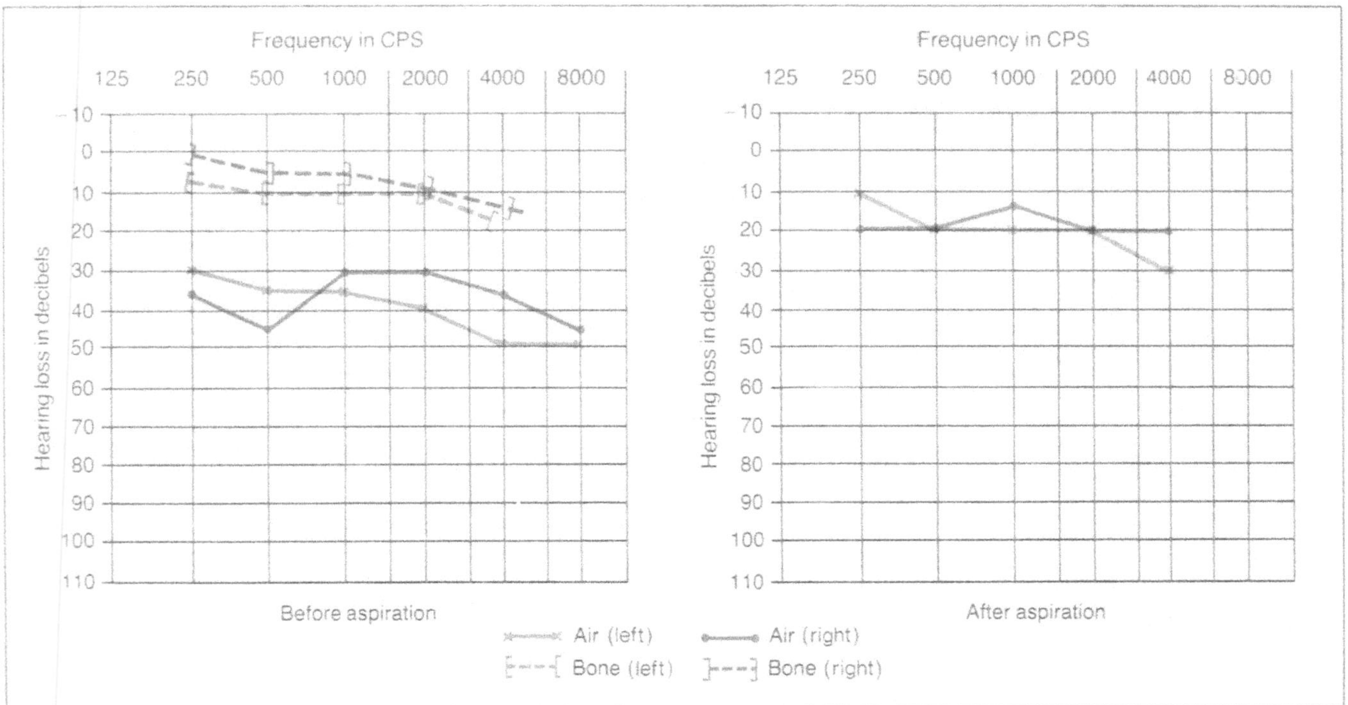

Figure 4.2. *The audiogram of a child with secretory otitis before (left) and after (right) aspiration of the ears, showing considerable immediate improvement in the conductive deafness.*

Throat Problems

Sore Throats

Infections in which the pharynx is the primary site of involvement are uncommon under the age of two years and reach a peak incidence from four to seven years. The use of the term 'tonsillitis' to describe all such infections probably contributes to the common misunderstanding about the importance of the tonsils and it is often helpful to emphasize to parents that absence of the tonsils fails to affect the frequency or the course of pharyngeal infections. Acute pharyngitis is most commonly caused by viruses but in a considerable proportion of cases, probably one third, is due to the group A beta-haemolytic streptococcus (Figure 4.3) (Ross et al. 1971). Other infections in which pharyngitis may be prominent include glandular fever (Figure 4.4), diphtheria and herpangina. It is not possible to distinguish clinically between viral and bacterial infections. However, the former tend to be associated with other 'viral' symptoms such as rhinitis and laryngitis and to be gradual in onset with only moderate fever, constitutional upset and pharyngeal inflammation; their total duration is usually less than five days. Streptococcal infections, on the other hand, are characterized by acute onset, high fever, constitutional symptoms including vomiting and diarrhoea, severe local pain, exudative tonsillitis and enlarged, tender cervical glands; the illness may last up to two weeks.

Treatment

The treatment is straightforward. If possible, a throat swab should be taken and then penicillin given either parenterally or orally. Wide spectrum antibiotics such as ampicillin are not indicated and this particular drug should be avoided as it gives a very high incidence of skin rashes in children with glandular fever. When streptococcal infection is confirmed, penicillin should be given for a full 10 days to prevent relapse. Erythromycin is probably the drug of choice in children who are sensitive to penicillin. An analgesic and antipyretic may

Figure 4.3. *This child presented with a sore throat before developing the typical rash of scarlet fever, which characteristically blanches with pressure.*

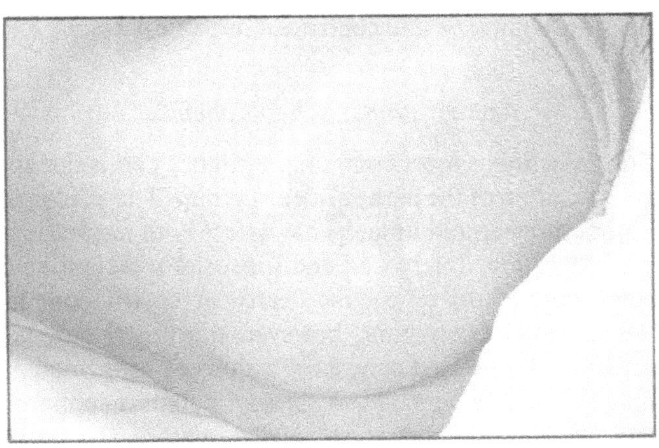

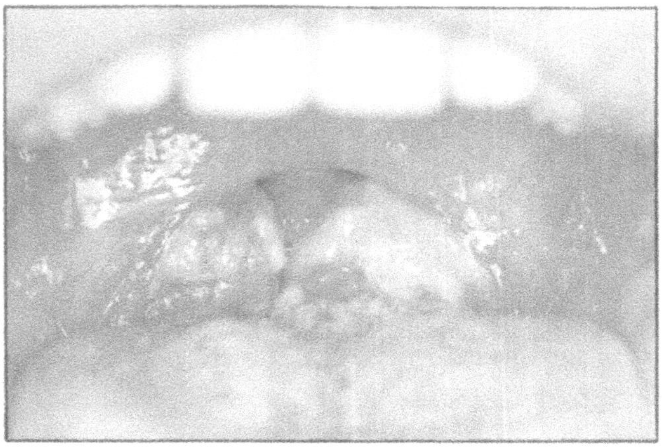

Figure 4.4. *Tonsillitis with a heavy exudate; streptococcal disease, glandular fever or diphtheria? In this case glandular fever.*

be needed; soluble aspirin may be gargled then swallowed. Complications of streptococcal sore throat include otitis media, peritonsillar or retropharyngeal abscess, acute glomerulonephritis and rheumatic fever, but fortunately all except the first are now uncommon.

Stridor

The chief causes of stridor, acute and chronic, are listed in Table 4.1. In any child with noisy breathing it is useful to observe the timing of the sound which may be inspiratory, expiratory or both. In children with chronic stridor a purely inspiratory sound usually arises above or at the level of the larynx and is less likely to be of serious import than expiratory, or combined inspiratory and expiratory stridor which often indicates a tracheal lesion (Figure 4.5). If the voice is hoarse or weak the larynx is likely to be involved but if it is muffled supraglottic tissues are probably at fault. Chronic upper airway obstruction from any cause may result in the development of cor pulmonale (Figure 4.6). Acute stridor, often called croup, is usually due to upper respiratory tract infection. There are two chief syndromes between which it is important to distinguish—acute laryngotracheobronchitis and acute epiglottitis. They are compared and contrasted in Table 4.2.

Acute Laryngotracheobronchitis

This infection is most common in infancy and is due to viruses, often of the para-influenza group. The stridor is at first inspiratory but later may affect both inspiration and expiration. Intercostal and subcostal recession and respiratory effort reflect the degree of obstruction. If the air entry is very poor, however, the stridor may be unimpressive and a diagnosis of asthma or bronchiolitis may mistakenly be made. A 'brassy' cough is common and the voice is characteristically hoarse. The most

Table 4.1. Causes of stridor.

Acute	Chronic
Laryngotracheobronchitis	Congenital laryngeal stridor
Epiglottitis	Micrognathia
Foreign body	Foreign body (Figure 4.5)
Retropharyngeal abscess	Vocal cord paralysis
Trauma	Laryngeal lesions
Angio-oedema	Vascular ring
Hypocalcaemia	Subglottic stenosis
Diphtheria	Tracheal lesions

Table 4.2. Clinical features of laryngotracheobronchitis and acute epiglottitis.

	Laryngotracheo-bronchitis	Epiglottitis
Age	3 months–3 years	3–7 years
Duration of illness	Days	Hours
Fever	Nil–moderate	High
Dysphagia sore throat	No	Yes
Dribbling	No	Yes
Voice	Hoarse	Muffled
Pathogen	Para-influenza virus	*Haemophilus influenzae*
Treatment	Maintain airway (intervention rarely required)	Maintain airway (endotracheal tube or tracheostomy usually required)
	Humidification	Parenteral ampicillin or chloramphenicol

Figure 4.5. *A foreign body must always be excluded as a cause of obstructive symptoms. This child's puzzling dysphagia and dyspnoea proved to be due to a coin stuck in the upper oesophagus.*

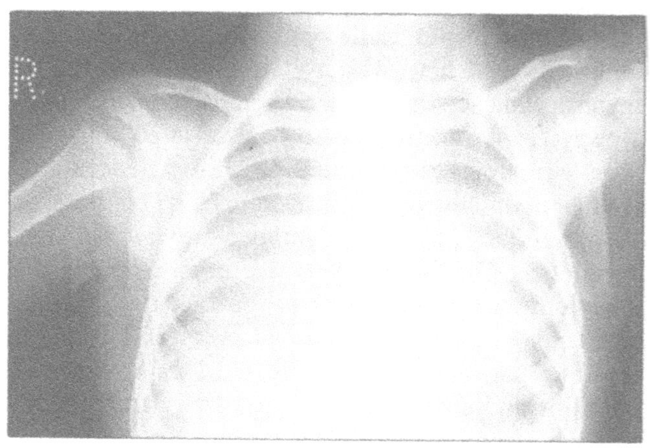

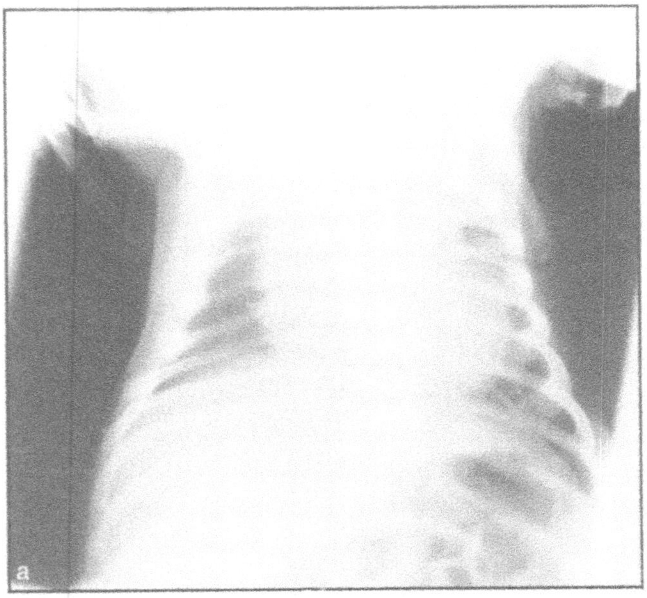

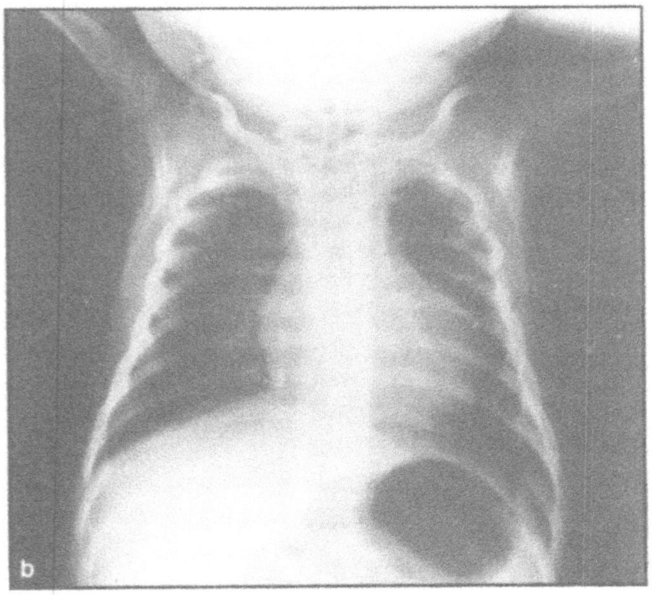

Figure 4.6. *This child with severe congenital laryngeal stridor developed cor pulmonale with an enlarged heart and congested lungs (a) which resolved rapidly after tracheotomy (b).*

important measure is careful observation in hospital for all but the mildest cases. If there is progressive dyspnoea with a rising pulse rate and irritability due to hypoxia, and especially if the pCO_2 is rising, establishment of an artificial airway by intubation of the larynx or tracheotomy must be considered. Humidified oxygen should be given as necessary. The humidity is soothing and helps avoid dryness of the upper airways. Antibiotics have no place in treatment and steroids, which have been recommended in order to reduce the swelling of upper respiratory tract tissues, are not of proven value.

Acute Epiglottitis

This dangerous acute infection generally affects children in the middle of their first decade and is typically due to *Haemophilus influenzae* type B, although other pathogens, such as pneumococci and group A streptococci, may be responsible (see *Lancet* 1978). The infection particularly affects the epiglottis and surrounding tissues, which become greatly swollen. The onset of the illness is rapid with fever, malaise, sore throat and progressive inspiratory stridor. The child presents a characteristic and distressing picture; he sits upright, leaning forward and looks (justifiably) anxious; he is 'toxic' and severely dyspnoeic with a harsh low-pitched stridor and he dribbles saliva from his open mouth. In the seriously ill child it is vital that the tongue is not depressed in an attempt to see the swollen cherry-like epiglottis because this can precipitate complete airway obstruction. He must be transferred immediately to hospital. It is reasonable to give a dose of parenteral ampicillin or chloramphenicol as long as this does not delay transfer. If complete obstruction occurs outside the hospital, emergency tracheotomy or puncture of the cricothyroid membrane offers the only hope of survival (figure 15.2, p 109).

Congenital Laryngeal Stridor

This is by far the commonest cause of chronic stridor in infants. It has also been called laryngomalacia and is usually due to collapse of the soft supralaryngeal and laryngeal tissues during inspiration. The onset of stridor usually occurs shortly after birth, progresses for the first few months of life, remains static during the latter half of the first year then gradually improves and resolves by 18 months to two years. The stridor is inspiratory and tends to be very variable, almost disappearing at rest but much aggravated by crying. If there is any doubt about the diagnosis, laryngoscopy is indicated to exclude other remediable lesions and a barium swallow to exclude a vascular ring. Most affected children make good progress but feeding difficulties and cyanotic attacks may occur and the stridor may be aggravated by upper respiratory tract infection. Occasionally tracheotomy is necessary (see Figure 4.6).

Tonsillectomy and Adenoidectomy

Finally, a word on the debatable matter of these operations. Discussion of the indications for them and their value continues to provoke more or less cheerful controversy between ENT surgeons, general practitioners, paediatricians, parents, journalists and everyone else who cares to enter the ring! We cannot improve on the

Table 4.3. Indications and contraindications for tonsillectomy and adenoidectomy (From Davis 1968, with permission).

Indications for tonsillectomy:

Quinsy that does not resolve completely on antibiotic therapy

Some cases of tuberculous cervical adenitis

'Carriage' of diphtheria (and in certain circumstances of β haemolytic streptococci unresponsive to antibiotics)

Sore throats associated with tonsillar remnants

Indications for adenoidectomy:

Recurrent suppurative or catarrhal otitis media with deafness and enlarged adenoids

Indications for tonsillectomy and adenoidectomy:

Evidence of right heart strain due to respiratory obstruction by enlarged adenoids

Conditions in which removal of the tonsils and/or adenoids should be considered:

Tonsils:

Recurrent tonsillitis of any frequency especially in the younger or older age-groups (3-6 or 9 on) (It has been shown that there is a lower incidence in the year or two after operation in young children)

Adenoids:

Prolonged postnasal obstruction with anorexia, snoring, intermittent deafness, cough due to true mouth breathing and presence of enlarged posterior cervical lymph nodes (here one should ask whether the objections to the child's symptoms are medical or aesthetic and whether they are his own or other people's)

Conditions that are not favourably influenced by tonsillectomy and/or adenoidectomy:

Frequent colds

Asthma

Rheumatic fever

Nephritis

Failure to thrive

Anaemia

Low IQ not related to deafness

Lack of *joie de vivre*

Ill health ascribed to 'focal sepsis'

Bronchiectasis

Relative contraindications to tonsillectomy:

Personal or family history of bleeding disorder

Emotional disturbance

Extreme youth

Lymphoma of tonsil

Relative contraindications to adenoidectomy:

Personal or family history of bleeding disorder

Emotional disturbance

Extreme youth

History of cleft palate followed by speech difficulties (here removal of adenoids may prevent palatal occlusion of postnasal space during phonation)

Table 4.4. Hazards of tonsillectomy and adenoidectomy (from Davis 1968, with permission).

Anaesthetic death (the procedure should not be carried out except under the supervision of a trained and experienced paediatric anaesthetist and a child in a panic should not be sent to the theatre whatever the inconvenience)
Death from primary or secondary haemorrhage (here technique is important: the tonsils should in general be dissected out, not guillotined and Denis Browne's vein must be identified if there is any bleeding. Routine bleeding and clotting tests may engender a false sense of security; it is the history, including the family history, that matters)
Operation in the presence of infection may result in secondary haemorrhage and should not be performed in these circumstances. Those in charge of the postoperative ward must be on the alert for insidious bleeding and ready to transfuse before irreversible shock is heralded by changes in pulse and blood pressure
Acute otitis media is a well known complication of the operation and should be sought for and treated with antibiotics when earache supervenes
Carotid thrombosis is a complication of removing the tonsils as well as of leaving infected tonsils alone
Vomiting and aspiration during the operation can lead to chronic pulmonary disease
The operation is sometimes followed by intractable obesity
The operation may initiate severe emotional disturbance of some duration. This is at least partly preventable by admitting mothers with their children whatever the inconvenience this may cause
Some asthmatic children actually become worse after removal of tonsils and adenoids and the operation should therefore be avoided as a symptomatic treatment for allergic rhinitis
Removal of the adenoids may be followed by speech disorder due to nasal escape with failure of palatal occlusion during phonation

summaries of the indications and contraindications (Table 4.3) and the hazards (Table 4.4) published by Davis in 1968.

References

Davis, J. A., *Medical News Magazine,* Suppl. Paediatrics, July 1968, p 16.

Lancet, 1978, **i**, 1294.

Ross, P. W., Chisty, S. M. K. and Knox, J. D. E., *Br. Med. J.,* 1971, **2**, 624.

Stott, N. C. H., *Br. Med. J.,* 1979, **1**, 29.

Further Reading

Birrell, J. F., *Paediatric Otolaryngology,* John Wright, Bristol, 1978.

Hughes, J. R. (Ed.), *Upper Respiratory Tract Conditions in Childhood,* Report of the 4th Ross roundtable on critical approaches to common paediatric problems, Ross Laboratories, Columbus, Ohio, USA, 1974.

5. Lower Respiratory Tract Problems

No doctor working with children needs to be reminded that lower respiratory tract infection is very common in childhood, but it is easy to forget how serious a problem it is. Although there has been a greater than tenfold reduction in childhood deaths from respiratory tract infection in the last 30 years, it remains a major killer, accounting for approximately one quarter of all deaths in childhood after the neonatal period. Since our national infant and child mortality rates compare unfavourably with those of several other countries in Western Europe, it is reasonable to conclude that improvement in the death rate from respiratory tract infection could be achieved.

Before discussing specific disease entities, several general points should be stressed.

1. The majority of lower, as well as upper, respiratory tract infections in childhood are caused by viruses. Bacterial infection usually causes serious disease with major systemic as well as respiratory symptoms and signs.

2. Hypoxaemia is common in serious pulmonary disease and oxygen therapy may therefore be life-saving. Normal children are always CO_2 sensitive, so high ambient oxygen concentrations may be given without fear of respiratory depression.

3. Physical signs in the chest are extremely difficult to elicit and interpret in children. It is especially easy to misinterpret conducted sounds from the upper respiratory tract as originating in the lungs. Most infants described as 'chesty' are, in fact, more accurately 'throaty'. Consolidation has to be massive before dullness to percussion is apparent, although pleural effusion, which is rare in children, can usually be detected. Many infants who are very ill have few signs in the chest and little to be seen on x-ray.

4. In seriously ill children a microbiological diagnosis must be made if possible. Sputum can rarely be obtained because children swallow it, but an attempt at a deep throat swab often provokes a diagnostically useful cough. Blood culture is an important means of identifying infection and other methods, e.g. direct aspiration of the lung, may be necessary.

5. Many serious underlying problems, e.g. cystic fibrosis, congenital heart disease and immunodeficiency, greatly increase susceptibility to infection but are rare. Children who are immunosuppressed may have serious pulmonary infections, which are frequently atypical in their clinical manifestations, are caused by unusual pathogens and require full evaluation before treatment.

Classification

Lower respiratory tract infection may be classified according to the pathogen involved, the chief anatomical site of the disease, the radiographic findings, and in several other ways. In this discussion, however, respiratory illness will be divided into the two categories—mild and severe—which determine most clinical decisions and which are usually apparent at the first glance. Obviously, there are situations in which this somewhat simplistic classification may prove misleading and some of these will be considered briefly.

Mild Illness

Bronchitis/Mild Bronchopneumonia

Affected children have fever and cough, often associated with upper respiratory tract symptoms and slight general constitutional upset. Swallowed upper tract secretions and sputum may provoke vomiting, but a good fluid intake is maintained and there is no dehydration. Apart from a slight increase in respiratory rate, the symptoms and signs are those summarized in Table 5.1 (left hand column). Auscultation may reveal rhonchi and some crepitations, and conducted sounds from the upper tract are often audible. Wheezy bronchitis is considered below.

Table 5.1. Typical findings in mild and severe lower respiratory tract infection.

	Mild illness	Severe illness
Clinical impression	Well child	Ill child, 'toxic'
Fever	Nil to moderate	High
Cough	Usually dry	Usually wet ('brassy' in bronchiolitis)
Respiratory rate	Normal: 40 newborn 30 infant 20 child	Increased +20
Respiratory pattern	Normal	Distressed: intercostal recession, flared nostrils, accessory muscles working, grunting
Cyanosis	Absent	Present
Heart rate	Normal: 140 newborn 100 infant 80 child	Increased +20 to 30 ±cardiac failure
Physical signs	Rhonchi ±wheeze ±crepitations	Consolidation or generalized crepitations

Causal Agents

Microbiological studies have shown that this syndrome is due almost invariably to viruses, usually either the respiratory syncytial virus (RSV) or those of the influenza/parainfluenza group. In contrast to the situation in adults, there is no evidence to suggest that overgrowth of the normal bacterial flora in the lungs plays a part in the aetiology of bronchitis in children. Occasionally, organisms such as pneumococci or β haemolytic streptococci are isolated but it is doubtful whether they play a part in pathogenesis.

Treatment

Treatment can only be symptomatic. Antipyretics and occasionally antitussives may be useful. Antibiotics are not indicated since they have no influence on the course of the illness or the development of complications, and they may further complicate the picture by causing rashes and gastrointestinal symptoms.

Severe Illness

Seriously ill children show the symptoms and signs detailed in Table 5.1 (right hand column). The cough may be unimpressive but there is often a high fever or occasionally, in infants, hypothermia. There may be very little to find in the chest: it is most important to recognize that severe parenchymal lung disease may be present with remarkably little in the way of classical clinical signs. If signs are present they are usually significant, but their absence means little in a sick child. Much more can be inferred from the associated findings of tachypnoea, respiratory distress and cyanosis. Thus, in contrast to adults, the diagnosis of serious pneumonia in children is made from the end of the bed!

The more important diseases which cause this picture are considered below.

Bronchiolitis

Clinical Features

This condition, which is caused by the respiratory syncytial virus, occurs in infants under the age of one year, the majority of whom are under six months. It occurs in epidemics between January and March (Figure 5.1). Typically, all the features of severe lower respiratory tract infection summarized in Table 5.1 are present. It is of interest that the respiratory syncytial virus is seldom responsible for serious illness in the neonatal period or in children past infancy, then causing only mild upper respiratory tract infection or bronchitis. During the vulnerable months of life, however, certain ill-understood features of the infant's response to the virus (possibly related to deficient mucosal IgA, an atypical reaction to transplacentally acquired maternal IgG or an early manifestation of allergy) may result in an acute reaction of the terminal airways with bronchiolar oedema, luminal obstruction and distal air-trapping.

The illness starts with symptoms of upper respiratory tract infection but within 48 hours has gone 'down onto the chest'. The infant becomes severely dyspnoeic and develops a repetitive hacking cough. His distress and restlessness increase as he becomes hypoxaemic. Marked tachycardia is present and about five per cent of infants develop heart failure. The signs in the chest are often obscured by coughs, rattles and grunts, but generalized high-pitched crepitations are characteristic. The chest radiograph shows marked overexpansion and sometimes patchy exudates (Figure 5.2).

Diagnosis

The clinical features of the illness are highly characteristic and, especially in epidemics, it may be inferred that RSV is almost certainly the culprit. Confirmation of the diagnosis within hours can, however, be obtained by the technique of immunofluorescence. The virus is present on the walls of cells from nasopharyngeal secretions and will take up antibody raised against RSV in rabbits. Fluorescein-labelled antibody to rabbit immunoglobulin

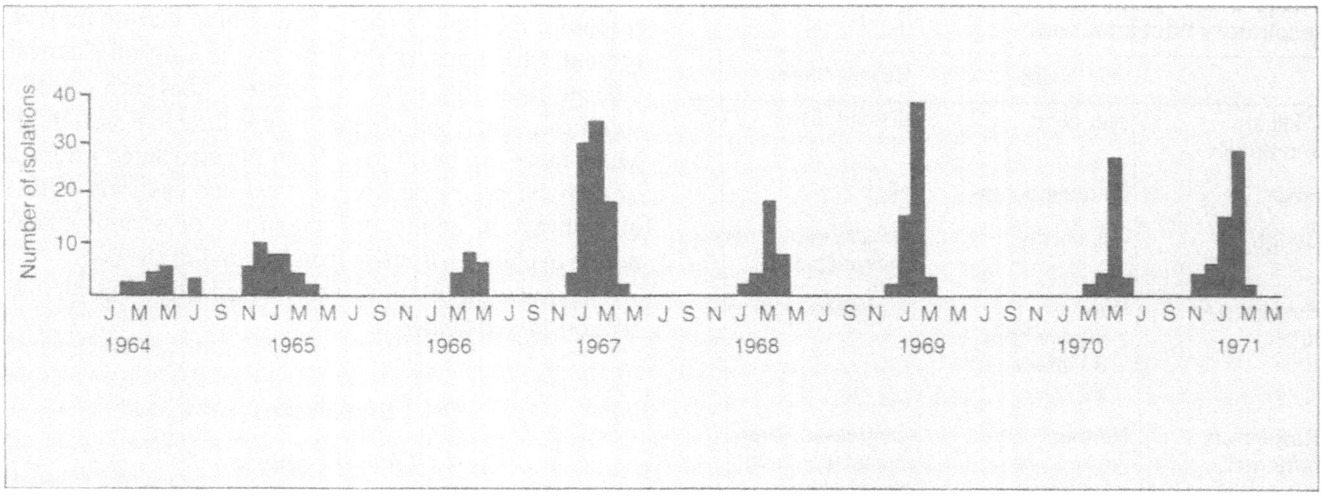

Figure 5.1. *Number of isolations of RSV according to month from children with lower respiratory tract illnesses (from Glezen and Denny 1973, with permission).*

is then used to mark these cells and is detected by fluorescent microscopy.

Treatment

Admission to hospital is required for all but the mildest cases. The aim of treatment is to support the infant until spontaneous recovery occurs. Oxygen is given, humidified and in sufficient concentration to keep the arterial oxygen tension greater than 8 kPa (60 mm Hg). If hypoxaemia cannot be relieved and/or CO_2 retention occurs, then ventilatory assistance with continuous positive airway pressure or intermittent positive pressure ventilation may be needed. Due to fever, hyperventilation and decreased intake, these infants are often dehydrated. They are unable to bottle feed and when really ill should not be tube fed because the nasogastric tube obstructs one nostril and increases the work of breathing, and a full stomach splints the diaphragm. Intravenous fluids should therefore be given to supply water, electrolytes and glucose. Diuretics may be needed if cardiac failure occurs. Bronchodilating drugs, such as adrenergic agents and methylxanthines, are of no value. Controlled trials have shown no definite benefit from steroid therapy, but it may possibly tip the balance favourably in difficult situations when, for example, the need for artificial ventilation threatens. Antibiotics have no place in treatment but most paediatricians prefer to give antibiotic cover to severely ill infants until the diagnosis is confirmed.

Figure 5.2. *Overdistended lungs with some right upper zone consolidation in an infant aged six months with bronchiolitis.*

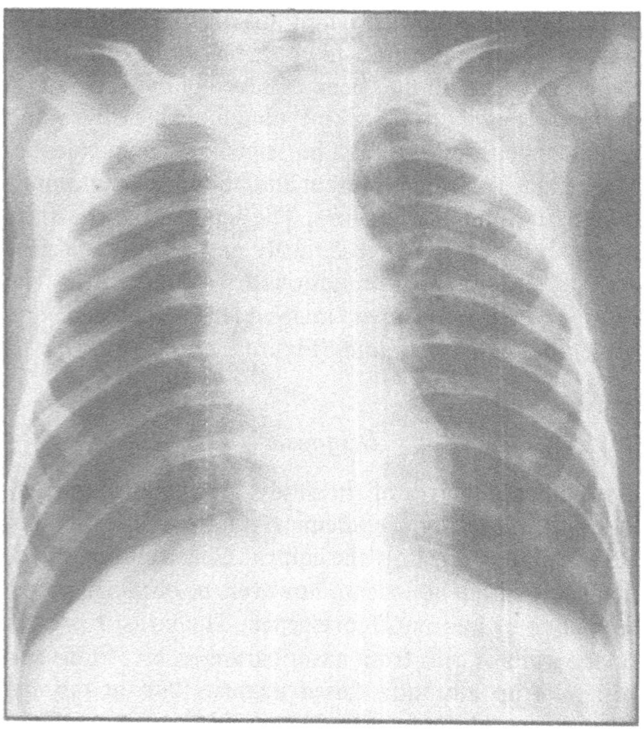

Natural History

The disease is usually of about 10 days duration and leaves no lasting sequelae. However, there is an increased incidence of subsequent wheezy bronchitis and asthma, especially in children who had attacks of 'bronchiolitis' in infancy without demonstrable RSV infection. It seems probable that such attacks simply indicate an asthmatic diathesis and do not themselves predispose to the later development of wheeziness.

Staphylococcal Lung Disease

Clinical Features

Children with staphylococcal lung disease are usually very ill and obviously require admission to hospital.

(Conversely, children well enough to stay at home are most unlikely to have staphylococcal disease.) In infants it may be difficult clinically to separate staphylococcal pneumonia from bronchiolitis. However, clues suggesting staphylococcal pneumonia include a preceding viral illness, another site of staphylococcal infection, such as boils, impetigo or a cervical abscess, and although the signs in the chest are very variable, consolidation is usually present on the chest x-ray.

Diagnosis and Treatment

The white cell count is usually greatly elevated but occasionally depression of the neutrophil count with toxic granulation is seen. Staphylococci may be seen on Gram stain of aspirates from the respiratory tract or sputum and may be cultured from these, and from the blood. The chest radiograph in staphylococcal pneumonia shows widespread consolidation which usually does not follow a clear lobar distribution (Figure 5.3). This emphasizes the important general point that all children with signs of severe parenchymal lung disease need a chest x-ray. When consolidation is shown, staphylococcal infection must be assumed present until proved absent. Treatment must therefore include intravenous administration of a penicillinase-resistant penicillin, e.g. flucloxacillin, in full dosage. The only deaths occurring in normal children in an MRC/PHLS survey of respiratory infection were due to staphylococcal pneumonia in those who had not been treated with a penicillinase-resistant penicillin (Court 1973).

Figure 5.3. *Extensive staphylococcal pneumonia, chiefly involving the right lung, in a three-year-old girl whose illness followed influenza. In spite of massive doses of appropriate antibiotics and all resuscitative measures, she died eight hours after this radiograph was taken.*

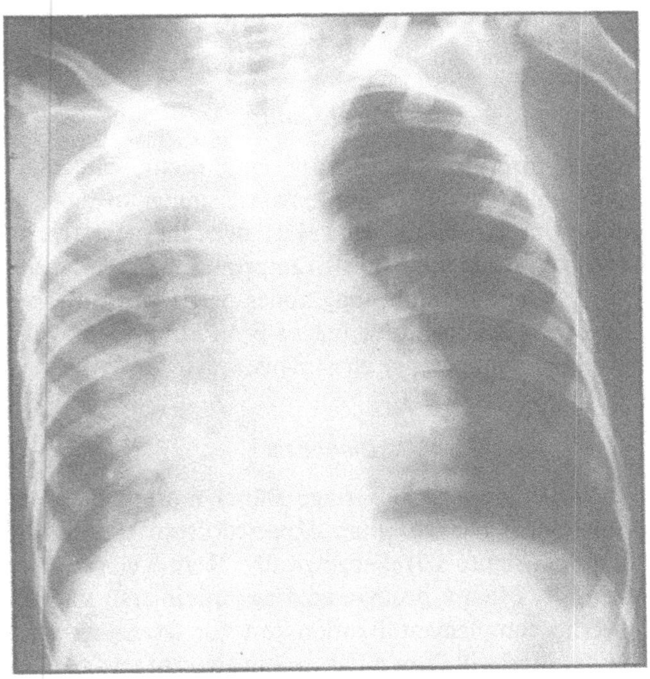

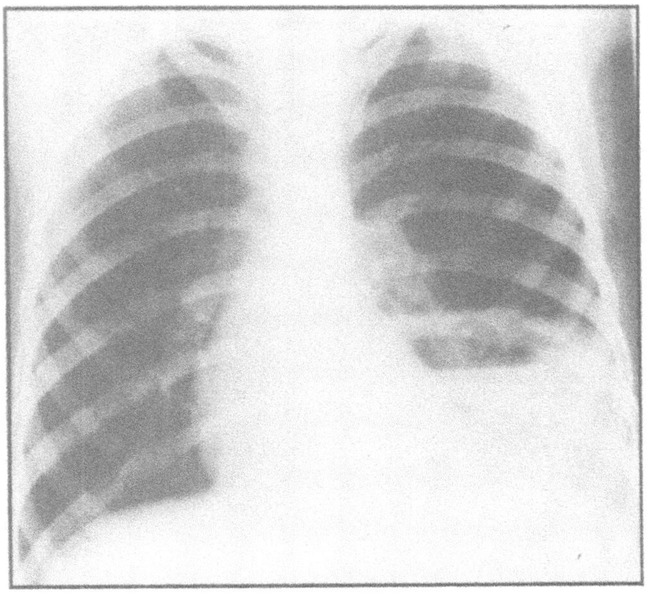

Figure 5.4. *A large abscess showing an air-fluid level in the left lung of a six-year-old girl recovering from staphylococcal pneumonia.*

Natural History

The course of the disease may be protracted. Oxygen and general supportive therapy are given as described for bronchiolitis. The child may develop a wide range of complications including lung abscess (Figure 5.4), empyema and pneumatoceles. However, these are treatable and provided that the correct antibiotic is given early enough the child should survive.

Pneumococcal Pneumonia

Clinical Features

The pneumococcus remains the major cause of lobar pneumonia in older children. The signs are those of severe pneumonia with high fever and sometimes delirium. In older children it is often possible to demonstrate an area of consolidation with decreased percussion note and bronchial breathing.

Diagnosis

The white cell count is raised with a marked neutrophilia, and pneumococci can be cultured from the throat swab, sputum and sometimes the blood. The chest radiograph is usually diagnostic, showing typical precise lobar segmental consolidation (Figure 5.5).

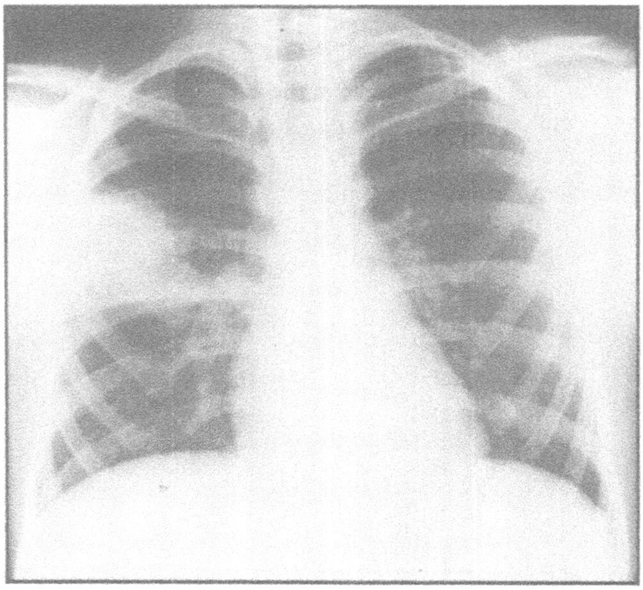

Figure 5.5. *Right upper lobar consolidation in a 10-year-old boy with pneumococcal pneumonia.*

Treatment

Many children have septicaemia and intravenous penicillin G in full dosage is the drug of choice. Broad spectrum antibiotics are less effective against the pneumococcus. If there is any suspicion whatever, based on the chest x-ray, the presence of other foci of infection, or indeed on any grounds, that staphylococcal pneumonia could be present then flucloxacillin should be given concurrently with the penicillin.

Infection Due to Gram-Negative Organisms

Haemophilus influenzae is a common commensal in the upper respiratory tract of children, and is often isolated from the throat or sputum of children with lower respiratory tract infections. Only rarely, however, is it the primary pathogen causing pneumonia and such children are severely ill. It is therefore not necessary to give an antibiotic to cover this organism in children with mild disease.

Other Gram-negative pathogens, e.g. *E. coli, Klebsiella, Proteus* and *Pseudomonas,* are very rarely encountered as pulmonary pathogens after the neonatal period except in immunocompromised children. Nevertheless, in seriously ill children in hospital with consolidation on chest x-ray, it is wise to add an anti-Gram-negative antibiotic, such as gentamicin, until a firm bacterial diagnosis is made. The combination of flucloxacillin and gentamicin is well tried and effective.

Exceptions to the Rules

A number of situations exist which do not conform to the above simple rules.

Wheezy Bronchitis

Perhaps as many as 15 per cent of infants have episodes of bronchitis and/or bronchiolitis in the first two years of life which are accompanied by definite wheeze, due largely to narrowing of the airways by mucosal oedema. This is discussed in detail in Chapter 6.

Foreign Body

The possibility of a foreign body must always be kept in mind when there is atypical respiratory tract disease in children (Blazer et al. 1980). The inhalation of a foreign body commonly presents as an acute choking episode in young children for whom hospital admission and bronchoscopy are mandatory. Older children may be well aware that they have inhaled something and require similar treatment. However, the problem often presents more subtly as persistent respiratory infection, associated with localized physical signs and radiological evidence of persistent collapse or consolidation in one pulmonary segment, which fails to respond to conventional therapy. Radiographic demonstration of partial collapse on inspiration but air-trapping on expiration is diagnostic (Figure 5.6). Bronchoscopy may be necessary to exclude this possibility with certainty.

Mycoplasma Pneumonia

Infection with *Mycoplasma pneumoniae* occurs in short epidemics every 18 to 24 months and sporadic cases are common.

Clinical Features

Severe forms of the disease may occur, but more commonly the initial symptoms are similar to those of mild viral bronchitis. However, over the next five to seven days the child fails to improve, the crepitations heard in one or more lung zones persist with marked listlessness and lassitude out of proportion to the mild fever and unimpressive chest signs.

Diagnosis

An x-ray taken at this stage shows more widespread radiological changes than expected from the clinical findings (Figure 5.7). Serologically, there is elevation of the ESR, often a positive cold agglutinin test, and the specific complement fixation test for *Mycoplasma* is positive and will show a rise in convalescent serum.

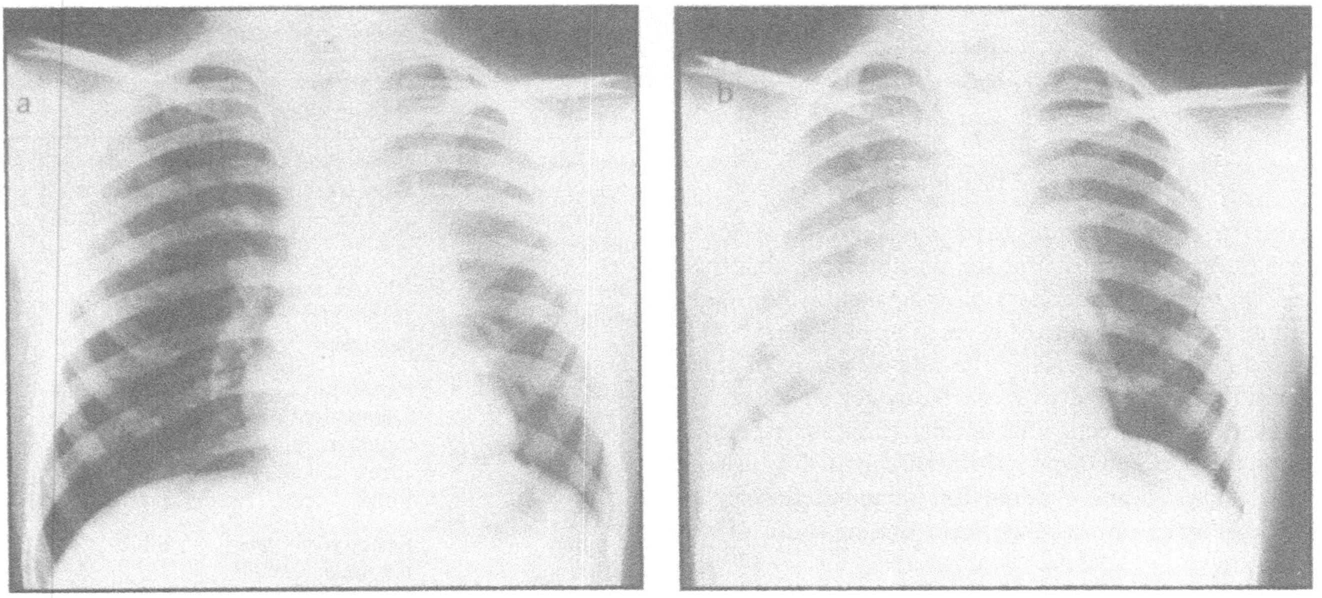

Figure 5.6. *a) Inspiration and b) expiration films of a five-year-old boy who had inhaled a peanut into the left main bronchus. On inspiration there is partial collapse and on expiration, air-trapping.*

Treatment

Erythromycin, given orally for 10 days, is the drug of choice in younger children. After the age of eight years tetracycline, which may be slightly more effective, can be given.

Tuberculosis

The incidence of tuberculosis varies with the size of the local immigrant population. In the UK, pulmonary TB in childhood is rare. However, this possibility must be considered in any child with unexplained persistent chest illness associated with radiological changes. The diagnosis can be checked initially by tuberculin testing and confirmed by identification of AFB in sputum or in early morning gastric lavage specimens. Recent evidence suggests that the Tine test is not a reliable skin test on such children and a formal Mantoux test using 0.1 ml of 1:1,000 tuberculin should be carried out.

Figure 5.7. *Extensive right-sided consolidation in a girl with Mycoplasma pneumonia who had fever, malaise and only trivial respiratory symptoms.*

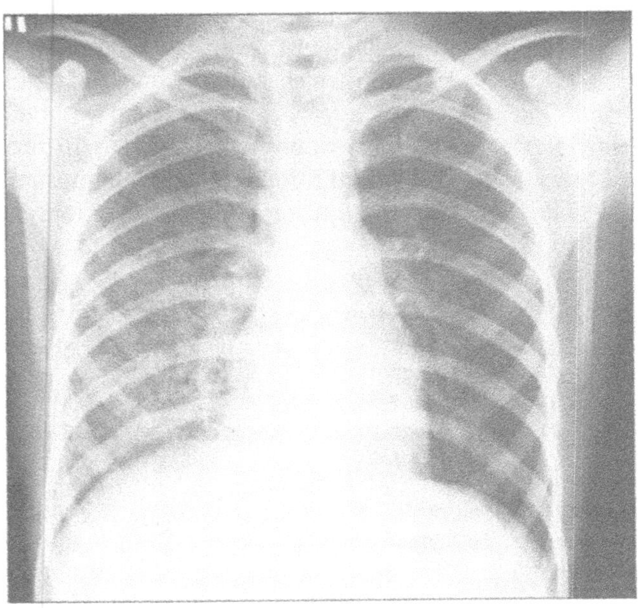

Pertussis

We have recently seen the worst epidemic of whooping cough for 20 years, due to the sharp fall in immunization rates which has resulted from the almost certainly unjustified adverse publicity (see chapter 2). In 1978, 66,000 cases and 11 deaths were notified. Affected children typically have paroxysms of coughing which culminate in either a prolonged inspiratory whoop or in collapse due to hypoxia. The disease is most severe, and mortality and morbidity greatest, in infants under six months of age. However, in older children symptoms—especially nocturnal paroxysms of coughing—may persist for several weeks.

Antibiotics probably play little part in relieving symptoms but they shorten the period of infectivity. Erythromycin is the drug of choice. Antitussives, antispasmodics and sedatives—in particular codeine—may be helpful in controlling the paroxysms in older children but in infants the important measures are close observation, good nursing care, restriction of stimuli to a minimum and tube feeding.

Problem Areas

Finally, we will consider two problems which are seen by all general practitioners.

Recurrent Chest Infection

When a child seems to have a real excess of lower respiratory tract infection, the possibility of abnormal susceptibility to pulmonary disease, such as a primary immunodeficiency state or cystic fibrosis (Figure 5.8) is raised. Table 5.2 indicates the relative rarity of these conditions compared with the frequency of lower respiratory tract infection in normal children, especially those from socially deprived environments. It is usually worth investigating children for immunodeficiency or cystic fibrosis only if they have one or more of the following:

1. Extremely frequent, severe or persistent lower respiratory tract infections.
2. Persistent unexplained radiological changes.
3. Other stigmata of disease, e.g. steatorrhoea, rectal prolapse or salty sweat.
4. Chest infections with significant failure to thrive.
5. A positive family history of relevant disease.

The Child with Chronic Cough

This symptom is rarely due to respiratory infection. The common causes are:

Figure 5.8. *Widespread reticular and nodular shadowing in both lung fields with thickening of the bronchial walls and overexpansion of the chest in a ten-year-old girl with cystic fibrosis.*

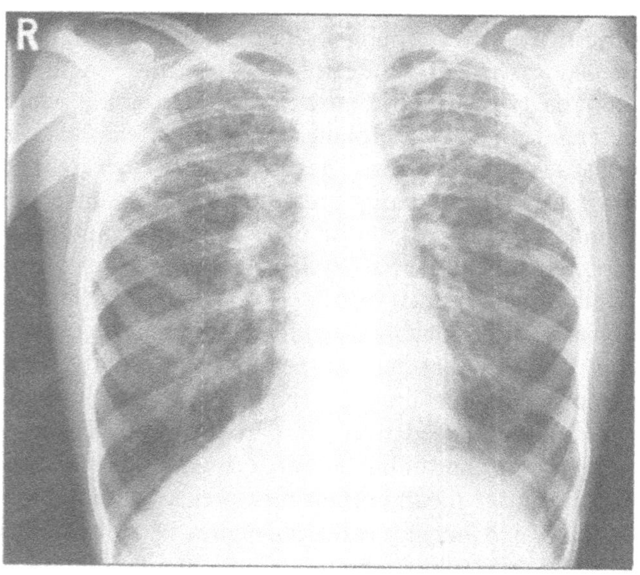

Table 5.2. Clinical features and incidence of conditions predisposing to lower respiratory tract infection.

Disease	Associated abnormalities	Approximate incidence
Viral infections of lower respiratory tract in normal children	None, child recovers within 10 days	All children at risk, 5-8 attacks per year common
Decreased secretory IgA	Attacks unusually severe and persistent	1:1000
Cystic fibrosis	Persistent pulmonary infection, loose stools, failure to thrive	1:2000
Immune deficiency syndrome	Sepsis elsewhere, diarrhoea, weight loss	1:5000

1. Asthma, especially nocturnal paroxysms of coughing.
2. Chronic postnasal drip (also worse at night), with rhinitis and sinusitis.
3. Pertussis and persistent postpertussis cough.
4. Tics, habit spasm, nervous cough.
5. Foreign body.

Summary

Lower respiratory tract infection is very common in childhood. The majority is viral in origin and viral disease may be assumed in children well enough to be managed at home. The most reliable signs of serious parenchymal lung disease are tachypnoea, respiratory distress and cyanosis; children showing these are likely to have bacterial disease which requires investigation, including an x-ray, and appropriate treatment without delay. Persistent physical or radiological signs in the chest raise the possibility of a foreign body, an unusual infective agent or increased susceptibility to infection.

References

Blazer, S., Naveh, Y. and Friedman, A., *Am. J. Dis. Child.*, 1980, **134**, 68.

Court, S. D. M., *Postgrad. Med. J.*, 1973, **49**, 812.

Glezen, W. P. and Denny, F. W., *New Engl. J. Med.*, 1973, **288**, 498.

Further Reading

Williams, H. E. and Phelan, P. D., *Respiratory Illness in Children*, Blackwell Scientific Publications, Oxford, 1975.

Wohl, M. E. B. and Chernick, V., *Am. Rev. Respir. Dis.*, 1978, **118**, 759-781.

6. Wheezy Children

WHEEZING is an extremely common symptom in childhood. It is defined in the Oxford English Dictionary as 'a whistling sound caused by difficult breathing'.

For clinical purposes it is useful to identify two major categories of wheezy children. In the first are children predisposed to asthma, which can be defined as an inherited tendency to develop bronchial wall oedema and bronchial muscular contraction when exposed to a wide variety of stimuli. Such children have increased bronchial lability, or bronchial hyper-reactivity, and comprise approximately 10 per cent of the child population. About half of these children have attacks of wheezing during childhood. The second category comprises children with non-asthmatic causes of extrinsic or intrinsic airways obstruction. These are listed in Table 6.1 and it is important to exclude them before concluding that a child who is wheezing for the first time has asthma.

Table 6.1. Non-asthmatic causes of wheezing in childhood.

Infection	Bronchiolitis
	Epiglottitis
	Laryngotracheobronchitis—croup
	Laryngitis
	Retropharyngeal or peritonsillar abscess
Cystic fibrosis	
Obstruction	Congenital laryngeal stridor and other laryngeal lesions
	Mucus in respiratory passages
	Extrinsic compression, e.g. lymph nodes (TB), tumour, foreign body in oesophagus
	Tracheal stenosis, bronchial stenosis
	Tracheomalacia, bronchomalacia
	Subglottic haemangioma
	Bronchopulmonary sequestration
Inhaled foreign body	
Vascular ring	
Post-neonatal ventilation—bronchopulmonary dysplasia	
Miscellaneous	Tetany
	Recurrent laryngeal nerve palsy
	Dislocation of cricoarytenoid joint

Wheezy Infants

Before discussing wheezy bronchitis and asthma we should mention briefly two varieties of wheezy illness peculiar to infants, which are often a prelude to asthma later in life.

Bronchiolitis

Bronchiolitis can be considered an idiosyncratic response to the respiratory syncitial virus in some infants. It was discussed fully in chapter 5 (page 41).

The Fat Happy Wheezer

This term was coined by Dr Peter Phelan of Melbourne to describe a well-recognized group of infants. Typically they are fat and between six and 15 months old. They wheeze and cough almost continuously, particularly at night, and yet they remain unperturbed, unlike their parents. In the surgery one is confronted by a beaming Falstaffian wheezy infant and one or more pallid dark-eyed parents! In spite of audible wheeze and widespread rhonchi the infant is afebrile and continues to feed with unabated enthusiasm. The chest radiograph is clear and none of the causes of wheezing listed in Table 6.1 is present. The wheeze is usually resistant to therapy: oral betamimetics have no effect and inhaled drugs are impractical. Some symptomatic relief may be obtained from drugs with a vasoconstrictor/decongestant action such as ephedrine or Actifed, and weight loss may help.

Do Wheezy Infants Develop Asthma?

The short answer is 'yes'. Follow-up studies after bronchiolitis show that virtually all affected infants have demonstrable abnormalities of bronchial lability on exercise and as many as 50 per cent may have further wheezing attacks later in life. The outcome for fat happy wheezers seems to be similar. Those particularly likely to have further trouble are infants who had 'bronchiolitis' but in whom no RSV was demonstrated, those with repeated attacks of wheezy illness and those with other evidence of atopic disease.

Wheezy Bronchitis

It is now recognized that wheezy bronchitis is part of the asthma spectrum so it is perhaps artificial to discuss it as a separate entity. Affected children and their first degree relatives often show evidence of an atopic diathesis. However, all general practitioners and paediatricians recognize a group of children between about 12 and 30 months of age who wheeze only in association with febrile illnesses. Such children at first seem to have simple bronchitis but, within 24 to 48 hours of the start of the illness, they become wheezy. This condition is caused by viruses and therefore antibiotics have no effect. The only drugs likely to be of benefit are bronchodilators but, unfortunately, these are ineffective in infants under 18 months, in whom the wheeze is due more to mucosal oedema than to bronchoconstriction.

Many children grow out of the tendency to infection-induced wheeziness but the longer they continue to have attacks the more likely they are to develop bronchospasm in response to other factors such as allergens, exercise or stress.

Asthma

There are four major types of stimuli which may provoke wheezing in children with increased bronchial lability:

1. Infections. These may be bacterial or viral; they evoke increased mucosal oedema and may release factors which provoke bronchoconstriction.

2. Inhalation of allergens. These combine with IgE and IgG in the bronchial mucosa and release active compounds which cause oedema and constriction.

3. Physical irritants or stimuli. These include exercise, inhaled irritants such as cigarette smoke, cold air or dust, laughing and coughing.

4. Psychogenic and emotional stimuli.

These factors may, of course, combine: a child might only wheeze if he ran (type 3 stimulus) away from home on a day with a high pollen count (type 2) after a fight with his mother (type 4) because she would not let him out to play when he had a cold (type 1)!

It is relatively easy to understand how antigen/antibody reactions can release biologically active substances causing oedema and constriction but more difficult to explain how other physical and emotional stimuli provoke wheeze. Current theories combine abnormalities in the control of the adenylcyclase/cyclic adenosine monophosphate (AMP) system in the cells lining the bronchi with autonomic nervous system imbalance. The final common pathway of bronchodilatation is through increased cyclic AMP in the bronchial smooth muscle cells. Bronchoconstriction may result if synthesis of cyclic AMP is compromised by decreased beta-adrenoreceptor activity, increased sensitivity to vagal activity or any other factor, and particularly if an antigen/antibody reaction occurs simultaneously.

Approximately one child in 20 has at least one asthmatic attack during his schooldays. However, although many of these continue to require occasional courses of bronchodilators and more have demonstrable abnormalities of bronchial function in response to exercise or provocation tests, no more than one in 10 will progress to serious asthma in adult life.

Aetiology

Asthmatic attacks are often of multifactorial aetiology, as emphasized above. An intercurrent viral infection, frequently with the rhinovirus, can be identified in about 25 per cent of attacks. When there is no prodromal illness and no associated fever, allergens, physical irritants, exercise and/or stress are usually involved and some idea of the contribution of each can be gained from the history.

The atopic group of diseases includes not only asthma but also eczema, hay fever, giant urticaria and food intolerance. Skin sensitivity tests in children with asthma show that the majority are sensitive to the house dust mite *(Dermatophagoides pteronyssinus)*, many respond to pollens (especially timothy grass) or animal danders (especially cats), and a small minority react to various other allergens, such as moulds. Demonstrable food allergy is rare.

Our personal practice is not to skin test most asthmatic children since sensitivity to the house dust mite can be assumed and a careful history often indicates other sensitivities. Skin tests may, however, be of help in convincing parents that their child really is allergic to animals. The British are extraordinarily reluctant to dispose of Tibbles or Rover—even when it is clear that they may provoke serious illness in their offspring. In this context it is often necessary to emphasize that sensitivity may arise after prolonged exposure to antigens. We frequently have to deal with the plaintive cry 'It can't possibly be Tibbles who causes the asthma, he has slept on Johnny's pillow for years'!

In vitro tests for specific antigens, such as the RAST (radioallergabsorbent) test, seem likely to prove of real value but we have little personal experience of these yet.

There is no doubt that psychogenic stress can provoke asthmatic attacks. Almost invariably, however, we find it more constructive to concentrate on good pharmacological control of the bronchospasm and to play down the emotional side. Once good control is established, many emotional problems simply disappear and psychiatric consultation need be considered only in children with persistent problems.

Diagnosis

In spite of the fact that asthma is so common, it is remarkably under-diagnosed. There seem to be three main reasons for this.

1. Mitigation of the symptoms by self-imposed avoidance measures. Asthmatic children soon become aware that many factors, especially exercise, make them breathless. They therefore avoid exertion and may in consequence be labelled 'lazy' and become withdrawn and unsociable children 'glued' to the television.

2. Failure to recognize asthmatic symptoms. This is especially true of nocturnal cough. Unless a child is recovering from whooping cough, persistent nocturnal cough should be ascribed to asthma until proved otherwise. Another common error is to attribute breathlessness on exercise to lack of fitness rather than to exercise-induced bronchoconstriction.

3. Reluctance to ascribe symptoms to asthma because of fear of this diagnosis. Many lay people still think of asthma as a crippling and largely untreatable condition. When making the diagnosis it is therefore most important to emphasize the good prognosis of childhood asthma with modern treatment.

When the diagnosis is clear on clinical grounds, the following tests may be helpful:

1. An eosinophil count. If this is raised it confirms the allergic nature of the disease.

2. A chest x-ray. This should be done to help exclude other diagnoses, to show whether any complication is present, such as right middle lobe collapse, and to indicate whether there is residual hyperinflation between attacks.

3. Skin tests. These may be useful in selected cases.

If the diagnosis is in any doubt, an exercise test should be performed. Ninety per cent of asthmatics, but no normal children, show a fall of at least 10 per cent in FEV_1 (or similar changes in other tests of airways resistance) after running for six to eight minutes. Running is a better provoking factor than other forms of exercise (Figure 6.1) and it now seems that the bronchospasm is due to hyperventilation with cool air (McFadden and Ingram 1979).

Treatment

Asthmatic attacks. The treatment of asthmatic attacks at home is described. The management of the severely ill child with status asthmaticus is beyond the scope of this book.

1. Beta-adrenergic drugs. These can be given orally, subcutaneously, intramuscularly, intravenously or by inhalation. Doses of salbutamol (Ventolin) and terbutaline (Bricanyl), the two drugs we personally favour, are shown in Table 6.2. Several other equivalent drugs are available; drug mixtures are undesirable. Salbutamol or terbutaline can be given prophylactically before asthma-inducing activities, intermittently to curtail a bout of wheezing, or given regularly to those with persistent symptoms. Four- to six-hourly doses should be given to a maximum of 20 to 50 ml of elixir or four to six tablets in 24 hours. Administration by inhalation is more effective. Older children can take eight to 10 puffs

Figure 6.1. *Changes in mean FEV_1 after different types of exercise (from Fitch and Morton 1971 with permission).*

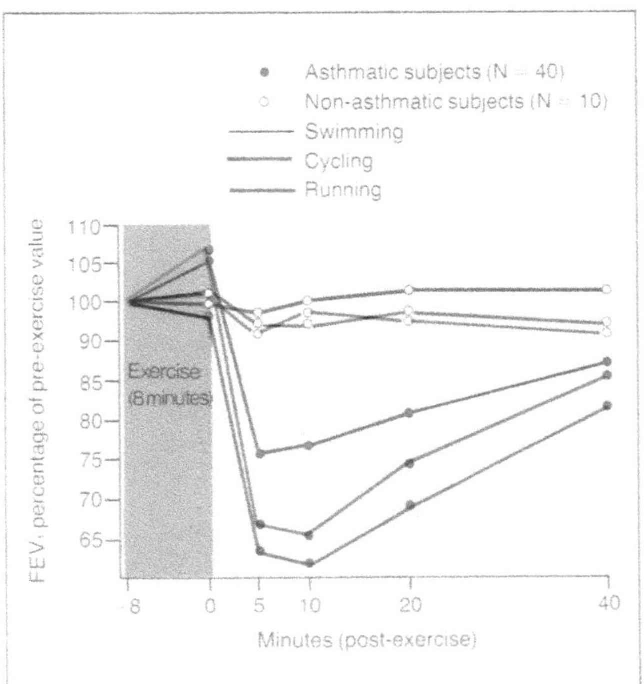

Table 6.2. Doses of beta-adrenergic bronchodilator drugs.

	Salbutamol (Ventolin)	Terbutaline (Bricanyl)
Elixir (5 ml)	2 mg	1.5 mg
Tablets	2 mg/4 mg	5 mg
Metered dose from pressurized aerosol	100 μg/puff	250 μg/puff
By inhalation from Rotahaler	200 μg/400 μg	–
Parenteral dose	8 μg/kg	10 μg/kg
Nebulizer solution	5-10 mg (1-2 ml)	5-10 mg (0.5-1.0 ml)

daily from an inhaler; it is important to check that they have mastered the technique. The nebulizer solution is equally effective and can often be used in younger children unable to manage an inhaler (Figure 6.2). Some children find Ventolin Rotacaps, which are inhaled by means of the Rotahaler, easier to use than a pressurized inhaler, especially if they are also using a Spinhaler for Intal. Children are also less likely to overdose themselves with this method of administration.

2. Intravenous aminophylline is highly effective in terminating acute attacks of asthma but it is potentially dangerous and should be given by slow intravenous injection in a dose of 5 mg/kg, ideally over 15 to 20 minutes.

3. Steroids. Intravenous hydrocortisone 100-200 mg should be given at home before transfer to hospital for severe asthmatic attacks which warrant admission. At least one hour is required for an effect to become apparent and several hours for major benefit. The use of steroids in perennial asthma is discussed below. They should not be used for mild intercurrent attacks or for wheezy bronchitis.

Sedatives, antihistamines and cough suppressants have no place in the treatment of asthmatic attacks because they are useless and, worse, may cause respiratory depression.

The perennial asthmatic. The first problem is to decide whether continuous therapy is necessary. It is clearly indicated for children who have persistent wheeze for more than two or three weeks which responds to bronchodilators but recurs when these are stopped. A more difficult problem is to decide when to start continuous therapy in children with intermittent bouts of asthma who are completely free of airways obstruction between the attacks. In this situation there are three rough guidelines we find helpful. Prophylactic treatment is likely to benefit children who turn up in the surgery or need home visits more than once a fortnight, require more than two absences from school per term or have more than two admissions to hospital per year.

It is important to emphasize that not only parents but also professionals, including nurses, health visitors and doctors, tend to underestimate the severity of asthma. For this reason objective criteria are useful. These include:

1. Growth. Height and weight are easily measured and children with chronic asthma are often underweight for height, a fact simply documented by plotting the measurements on centile charts. Severe and prolonged asthma may cause considerable stunting of growth. When the disease is controlled, remarkable catch-up growth may occur (Figure 6.3).

2. The chest shape. Persistent hyperinflation with an increased anteroposterior diameter and often a deep sulcus overlying the diaphragmatic attachment strongly suggests severe asthma (Figure 6.4). The changes are usually better seen on a chest radiograph which typically shows high shoulders, a transverse rib pattern, a flat-

Figure 6.2. *An 18-month-old child using a powered nebulizer.*

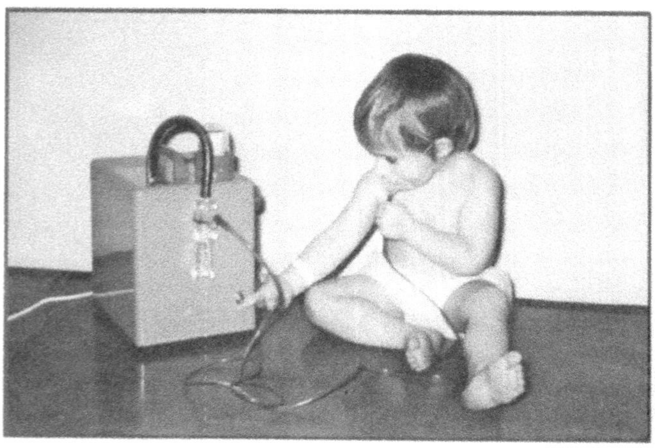

Figure 6.3. *Rapid catch-up of height and weight in a child with severe asthma after the disease was controlled (from Roberton 1977 with permission).*

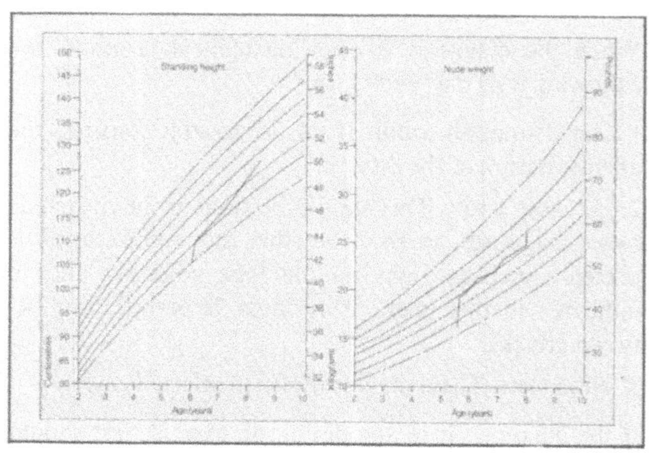

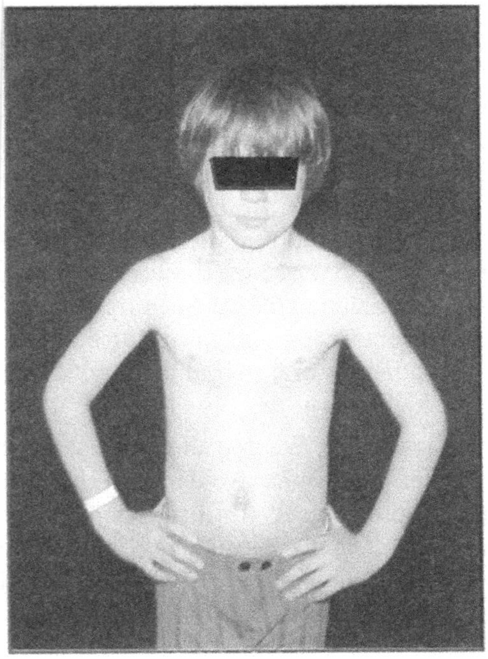

Figure 6.4. *An asthmatic boy showing the typical chest shape with over-inflation and a diaphragmatic (Harrison's) sulcus.*

tened diaphragm and more than nine ribs visible posteriorly (Figure 6.5). The increased anteroposterior diameter is apparent on a lateral film.

3. Peak flow measurements. These can be recorded regularly at home by the patient and entered in a diary. They offer the most accurate objective means of day-to-day assessment of airways resistance.

Treatment for the perennial asthmatic may include the following:

1. Beta-adrenergic drugs. These are most effective by inhalation but in children who are unable to manage inhalers they can be used continuously in elixir or tablet form in the doses shown in Table 6.2, given four to six times daily.

2. Theophylline preparations. Properly used these are highly effective and are justifiably regaining popularity. Dosage is critical and, ideally, blood levels should be checked. However, 20 mg/kg/24 hours of theophylline usually proves adequate for maintenance. If the drug is poorly tolerated it may be necessary to start at a lower dose. Preparations containing choline theophyllinate are only approximately 66 per cent theophylline by weight and those containing aminophylline 85 per cent theophylline, so appropriate dosage adjustments must be made to give 20 mg/kg/24 hours of theophylline. In general theophylline preparations have to be given six-hourly but the newer long-acting preparations allow for

Table 6.3. Theophylline preparations (recommended dose 20 mg/kg/24 hours of theophylline).

	Elixir (5 ml)	Tablets	Dose frequency
Choledyl (66% theophylline)	62.5 mg	100/200 mg	6 hourly
Etophylate (57% theophylline)	125 mg	250 mg	6 hourly
Phyllocontin (85% theophylline)	—	100/225 mg	12 hourly
Nuelin (pure theophylline)	60 mg	125 mg	6 hourly
Nuelin S.A.	—	175/250 mg	12 hourly
Rona-Phyllin (pure theophylline)	27.5 mg	100/200 mg	6 hourly
Rona-Slophyllin	—	60/125/250 mg	12 hourly

12 hourly therapy. Some convenient preparations are listed in Table 6.3. They can be combined usefully with the beta-mimetic drugs since their effects are additive.

3. Sodium cromoglycate (Intal). This compound prevents the antigen/antibody reaction which triggers the asthmatic process within the lungs. When starting a child on Intal it is important to emphasize four points to the parents:

a) The drug is a prophylactic and is of no value for treating acute attacks (there is no point, therefore, in using Intal Compound, plain Intal should always be prescribed).

b) It must be given at least three, and preferably four, times daily to be effective.

Figure 6.5. *Chest radiograph of severe asthmatic showing marked over-expansion of lungs.*

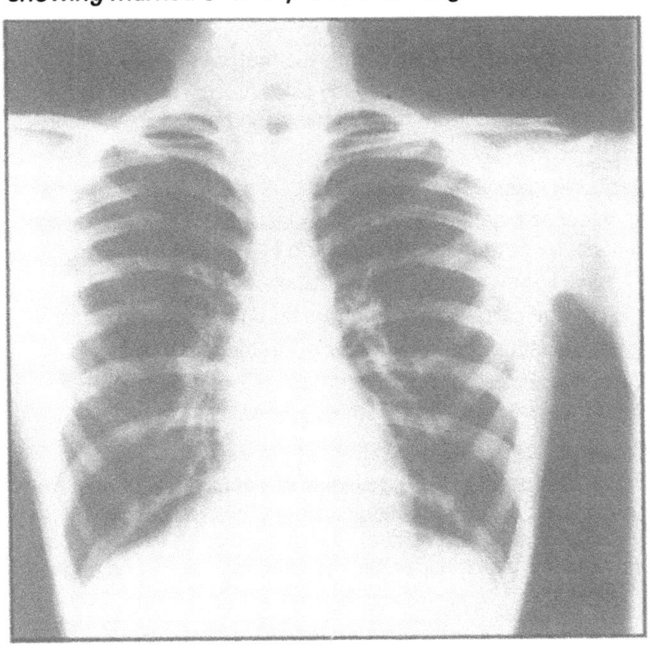

c) Before abandoning a trial of therapy, Intal should be given regularly for at least two, and preferably four, weeks while controlling intercurrent bronchospasm with other drugs, as necessary.

d) An extra capsule of Intal can be inhaled prophylactically before activities, such as exercise, which are likely to provoke bronchoconstriction.

In children unable to manage the Spinhaler, Intal nebulizer solution can be given with a power-operated nebulizer via a face-mask (Figure 6.2).

In perennial asthma, in addition to drugs given prophylactically, it is important to provide a means of treating breakthrough wheeze. Beta-mimetic drugs by inhalation are usually most effective, using the pressurized aerosol in older children and a nebulizer when necessary.

Approximately 75 per cent of children with perennial asthma can be satisfactorily controlled with regular Intal and a beta-mimetic drug for breakthrough wheeze.

4. Inhaled steroids. About 25 per cent of asthmatic children require inhaled steroids. Metered aerosols, either beclomethasone (Becotide 50 μg/puff) or betamethasone (Bextasol, 100 μg/puff) are used in six-hourly doses, giving from four to 16 puffs/day. If the child prefers the Rotahaler, Becotide Rotacaps can be used. It has been demonstrated recently that the larger doses cause adrenal suppression but growth failure has not been documented. However, it seems wise that children with asthma of sufficient severity to warrant steroid therapy should have hospital evaluation.

When using inhaled steroids, there is little extra benefit to be gained by continuing with Intal but, as usual, beta-mimetic drugs by inhalation should be given for breakthrough wheeze. In some children occasional, short, sharp courses of oral steroids, such as prednisolone 25, 20, 15, 10 and 5 mg on successive days, may abort serious asthmatic attacks. Such treatment clearly needs careful supervision and must not be allowed to shade into continuous oral steroid therapy, the dangers of which are well known.

5. Allergen avoidance. We give all perennial asthmatics instructions on house mite avoidance (Table 6.4) and tell them to avoid contact with furry animals, particularly those to which definite allergy is identified by history and/or skin testing. Avoidance of dietary allergens, including milk, seems only exceptionally to be of benefit.

6. Hyposensitization. In children who are strongly house-dust mite sensitive, hyposensitization has been shown recently to effect useful improvement but not elimination of symptoms.

Table 6.4. House mite avoidance measures.

Bedroom

Essential measures:

1. Remove feather pillows and eiderdowns—replace with ones having a synthetic filling
2. Thoroughly vacuum the mattress, the pillows and around the base of the bed or divan. Enclose the mattress top surface and sides in a plastic cover
3. Each day 'damp dust' the plastic mattress cover
4. Each week change and wash pillow cases, sheets and underblanket: vacuum the bed base and around the covered mattress

Desirable measures:

1. Woollen blankets should be replaced by nylon or 'terylene' quilts or by cotton cellular ones and be washed frequently
2. Have light washable curtains and wash frequently
3. Remove carpets and cover the floor with linoleum or vinyl
4. Use a vacuum cleaner with disposable paper bags

Note: If your child shares a bedroom *all* other beds in the room must be treated similarly

Other rooms

Particular attention should be directed at removal of dust from upholstered furniture (which harbours the type of dust to which your child is sensitive). Vacuum clean this furniture at least twice a week, especially the head rest, arms and edges of the seats

From Sarsfield et al. 1974.

Non-Asthmatic Causes of Wheezing in Childhood

Some of the more common problems listed in Table 6.1 are discussed in relation to upper and lower respiratory tract problems in chapters 4 and 5. A useful diagnostic point is the fact that in many of these conditions most noise is heard during inspiration, in contrast to true wheeze in which it is primarily heard in expiration. We will comment briefly on two conditions which can cause diagnostic problems. A third, cystic fibrosis, is discussed in greater detail in chapter 7.

Inhaled Foreign Body

An inhaled foreign body must be suspected in any child who has wheezing of sudden onset without the usual antecedents of asthma, especially if the wheeze is localized and started after an episode of coughing or choking. The condition can usually be diagnosed radiologically by demonstrating either air-trapping, where there is partial obstruction (see figure 5.6 page 45), or atelectasis, in complete obstruction, distal to the object. Inhaled foreign bodies must be removed by bronchoscopy without delay.

Vascular Ring

A constricting vascular ring should be considered in a child whose wheeziness started early in life, is associated with dysphagia and/or choking and fails to respond to antispasmodic therapy. The diagnosis is made by barium swallow and the treatment is surgical.

Conclusion

Fortunately, most of the conditions which may mimic asthma offer diagnostic clues to the alert physician. It is clearly important to bear in mind the words of Chevalier Jackson 'All that wheezes is not asthma'.

References

Fitch, K. D. and Morton, A. R., *Br. Med. J.*, 1971, **4**, 577.

McFadden, E. R. and Ingram, R. H., *New Engl. J. Med.*, 1979, **301**, 763.

Roberton, N. R. C., *The Asthmatic Child*, Fisons Ltd, Loughborough, 1977.

Sarsfield, J. K., Gowland, G., Toy, R. and Norman, A. L. E., *Arch. Dis. in Childh.*, 1974, **49**, 716.

7. Cystic Fibrosis

CYSTIC fibrosis (CF) is the commonest lethal autosomal recessive condition affecting the white population of the UK. The incidence is approximately 1 in 2,000, which implies a carrier rate of about 1 in 25. This high incidence indicates that the heterozygote carrier state may confer some biological advantage, but it is not known what this might be. The underlying biochemical defect has not been elucidated, but clinically it is useful to regard the disease as a disorder in which abnormally viscous mucus is produced which tends to obstruct the ductules of all body tissues that secrete it. Behind this obstruction, infection and fibrosis develop in involved organs.

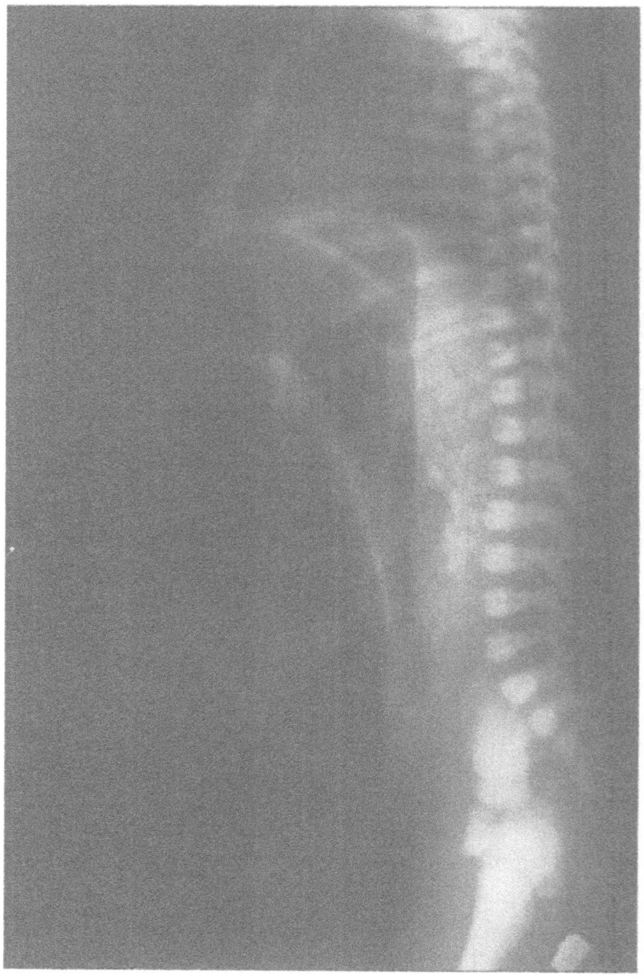

Figure 7.1. *Meconium ileus. Grossly dilated loops of small intestine with a virtual absence of fluid levels are seen in this lateral erect abdominal radiograph. No gas is visible in the pelvis. At operation the small intestine was obstructed by tenacious meconium. (Courtesy of Dr Malcolm Chiswick.)*

Diagnosis

The major impact of the disease is on the lungs and the gastrointestinal tract, and it usually presents in one of three ways:

1. Recurrent severe lower respiratory tract infection: in particular, infection with *Staph. aureus, Haemophilus influenzae,* and *Pseudomonas aeruginosa.*

2. Failure to thrive (see chapter 1) with malabsorption and steatorrhoea due to lack of pancreatic lipase. (Creatorrhoea, excessive loss of nitrogen in the stools, also occurs but is of much less clinical significance.)

3. Meconium ileus in the newborn: obstruction of the ileum by tenacious meconium which has not been digested in utero by pancreatic enzymes (Figure 7.1).

A child with any of these problems should have a sweat test. Localized sweating is induced in the skin by pilocarpine iontophoresis and the sodium content of the sweat, collected on filter paper, is measured. In patients with CF the sweat sodium usually exceeds 70 nmol/l, whereas in normal children, including heterozygotes, it rarely exceeds 30 nmol/l. Correctly performed the test is extremely reliable and discriminating.

The Lungs

The lung lesion of CF is a progressive chronic bronchitis which eventually causes emphysema, bronchiectasis and microabscesses (Figure 7.2), cor pulmonale develops sooner or later and is the cause of death in 90 per cent of patients.

Treatment

The aim of treatment is to retard the development of these changes. Useful measures include:

1. Regular chest physiotherapy. Postural drainage and percussion should be used at least once or twice per day, and as necessary when secretions are excessive.

2. Antibiotics. The use of antistaphylococcal antibiotics is particularly important. In advanced cases, with chronic *Pseudomonas* infection, inhalation of aminoglycoside antibiotics may also be used.

3. Antispasmodic medication. Although it is not confirmed that an excess of patients with CF have bronchospasm, 10 per cent of all children, including those with CF, have asthmatic symptoms at some time in childhood. If a child with CF is wheezing, a careful trial of bronchodilators should be undertaken.

4. Other measures. Patients should always be immunized against pertussis, measles and probably influenza, and they should receive BCG. Aspergillosis must be treated if it develops. Cor pulmonale should be treated with diuretics, digoxin is of doubtful benefit; once this complication has developed, however, the prognosis is poor and most patients die within a year.

There is dispute about the most effective combination of these measures but most paediatricians fully immunize children with CF, use antistaphylococcal antibiotics liberally and instruct parents in giving their children regular physiotherapy at home.

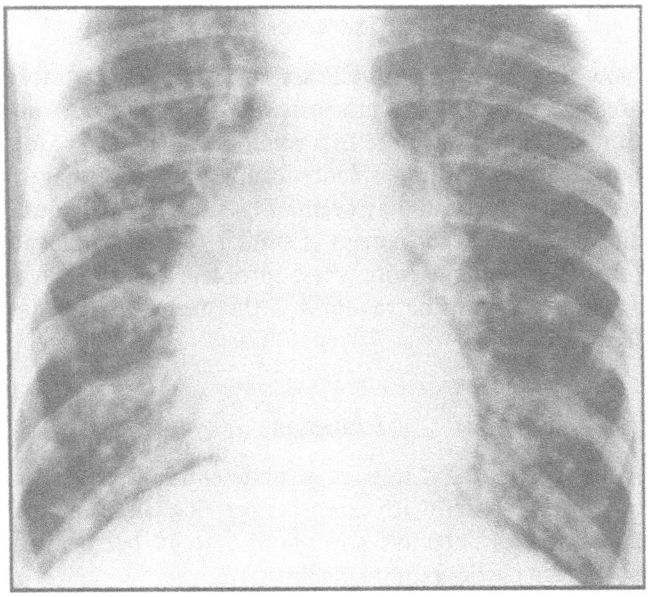

Figure 7.2. *Widespread reticular shadowing throughout both lung fields with nodular opacities in both lower lobes and thickening of the bronchial walls in a nine-year-old boy with cystic fibrosis.*

The Gut

Malabsorption

The deficiency of pancreatic enzymes causes malabsorption. To a large extent this can be controlled by the regular use of pancreatic supplements (Pancrex, Neutrazyme, Cotazym) which contain varying amounts of lipase, amylase and trypsin. These should be taken with every meal or snack. A low-fat diet may help patients with severe steatorrhoea, but most work out for themselves a diet which is reasonably palatable and with pancreatic supplements does not cause abdominal pain or excessive flatus or stool frequency. Except in rare cases there is no evidence that more complex elemental diets are of any benefit.

In the few children in whom large doses of pancreatic supplements and a careful diet fail to control the gut symptoms, regular oral alkalis or cimetidine can be given in addition to prevent gastric acid from breaking down the pancreatic supplements before they have an effect.

Abdominal Pain

Pain is usually due to subacute obstruction from thick inspissated gut contents, the 'meconium ileus equivalent'. It can usually be controlled by increasing the dose of pancreatic supplements and giving a mild laxative. In some cases, however, a wetting agent, acetylcysteine, given as an oral 10 per cent solution, may be useful.

Intussusception

The incidence of intussusception is increased in CF, and this possibility should be considered in a child with obstructive symptoms.

Rectal Prolapse

In malnourished, chronically coughing children with loose and frequent stools, the rectum may prolapse. Conservative treatment and measures to improve nutrition, the bowel habit and the chest are usually sufficient.

The Liver

Now that patients with CF are surviving longer, more are developing biliary cirrhosis due to biliary obstruction with tenacious bile. In a small proportion of cases, portal hypertension, splenomegaly and oesophageal varices develop and may eventually cause haematemesis and melaena. Management is similar to that employed for other patients with these problems. Porta-caval anastomosis may be required if the haemorrhages are frequent.

Diabetes

Although the main impact of pancreatic disease is on exocrine function, with extensive scarring islet function also becomes defective and about 5 to 10 per cent of adolescent cystics require insulin.

Other Problems

Nasal Polyps

Patients with CF have an increased incidence of nasal polyps: if symptomatic they should be removed.

Hyponatraemia

In hot weather, due to the high salt content of sweat, patients with CF may become severely hyponatraemic. Salt supplements should therefore be given.

Infertility

Due to atresia of the vasa deferentia, 98 per cent of male patients have azoospermia and are infertile.

Prognosis for Cystic Fibrosis

With the management outlined above, the outlook for children with CF has improved and about 75 per cent now reach their 18th birthday. There is some evidence, in males in particular, that the rate of progression of the disease then slows down.

Further Reading

Anderson, C. M., Cystic Fibrosis, in *Textbook of Paediatrics,* Forfar, J. O. and Arneil, G. C. (Eds), Churchill Livingstone, Edinburgh, 1978.

Chiswick, Malcolm, L., *Neonatal Medicine,* Update Books, London, 1978, p. 73.

8. Fits, Faints and Funny Turns

FITS and faints in children present problems familiar to all general practitioners and paediatricians. In a recent survey from the National Child Development Study it was reported that no less than 6.7 per cent of a large unselected sample of children had a history of seizures or other episodes of loss of consciousness by the age of 11 years (Ross et al. 1980). This is a rewarding area of paediatric medicine, both diagnostically and therapeutically, and one in which good clinical methods are often of more value than sophisticated investigative techniques.

Definitions

A useful working definition of a fit is 'an episodic alteration of consciousness and/or motor or sensory function due to inappropriate and uncontrolled discharge of cerebral neurones'. Such electrical discharges may be generalized or focal, isolated or recurrent, and primary (idiopathic epilepsy) or secondary (symptomatic epilepsy). A simple aetiological classification is given in Table 8.1.

Table 8.1. Types of fits occurring in childhood.

Chronic, recurrent
Low convulsive threshold
Idiopathic epilepsy
Organic epilepsy
Normal convulsive threshold
Febrile convulsions
Metabolic disturbance, e.g. hypoglycaemia
Acute, non-recurrent
Infection:
of CNS
extra-CNS
Hypoxia
Trauma
Metabolic
Mass lesion
Cerebrovascular accident
Others

Clinical Assessment

In the evaluation of these problems, however, the crucial diagnostic step is often the differentiation of true fits from the many conditions which may mimic them. This important distinction may be extremely difficult to make and it is worth emphasizing that, when uncertainty is present, it is always better to acknowledge it ('odd turns, ? type') than to attach even a provisional diagnosis ('probable fits') because of the tendency of a diagnostic label, however tentatively applied, to stick tenaciously once it has found its way into a patient's record.

Paediatrics is primarily concerned with the effects of disease processes on maturing individuals and, in this area as in so many others, children show a repertoire of responses largely determined by the stage of maturity reached. Age is a most important factor in determining the clinical pattern of fits and their equivalents. Table 8.2 indicates the frequent types of episodic attack which occur within various age ranges, and contrasts true fits with some of the conditions which may mimic them.

History Taking

The clinical assessment of the problem must begin with a detailed history obtained from family members. This route is lined with traps for the unwary. Important clues are easily missed, e.g. a family history of fits, details of the pregnancy and perinatal period, a previous head injury or an episode of illness suggesting meningitis or encephalitis. Since an attack can seldom be witnessed by the doctor and the relatives have often been too fright-

Table 8.2. Fits and other episodic attacks in children.

Typical age of onset	Fits	Faints and 'funny turns'
Less than 1 month	Incomplete grand mal Focal/multifocal	Jittery' infant Apnoeic spells
1 month to 6 months	Incomplete grand mal Infantile spasms	Breath-holding attacks Colic
6 months to 4 years	Febrile convulsions Astatic-myoclonic	Breath-holding attacks Infantile syncope (reflex anoxic seizures) Rigors Infantile masturbation
More than 4 years	Idiopathic grand mal Psychomotor Other focal Petit mal, atypical petit mal Astatic-myoclonic	Cardiovascular problems: vasovagal attacks arrhythmias Stokes-Adams attacks Functional disorders: simulated attacks hysteria habit spasms, sleep jerks, night terrors, overbreathing tetany Metabolic problems: hypoglycaemia hypocalcaemia Drug reactions: dystonic and dyskinetic reactions (Fentazin, Stemetil, Serenace, Maxolon, etc.) Migraine, periodic disorders Benign paroxysmal vertigo

ened to make close observations, it may take time and more than one interview to piece together an accurate account. It is also remarkable how often the 'wrong' relative brings the child to the doctor. Important matters to establish include:

1. In what circumstances do the attacks occur?
2. Are there any precipitating factors?
3. Is there a pattern?
4. Is there an aura or other premonitory symptom or sign?
5. What is the exact sequence of events?
6. Have simple observations on the state of consciousness, colour, pulse rate and focal signs been made during the attacks?
7. Is recovery immediate or delayed?
8. Is there sleepiness, headache, focal weakness or any other symptom after the attack?

Physical Examination

Physical examination is often negative but the absence of findings is in itself reassuring to the doctor, parent and patient. The degree of reassurance tends to be directly proportional to the thoroughness with which the search for clues has been made and such a search may prove rewarding. Many important physical signs are easily missed, e.g. a cerebral bruit, asymmetry of the child or the tendon reflexes, scarring of the tongue from biting, skin lesions (Figures 8.1 and 8.2), a cardiac irregularity—such a list could be extended indefinitely.

Tread with great care and even so be prepared suddenly to find yourself at the bottom of one of those traps for unwary doctors, where you can be sure of good company in your embarrassment, including that of the authors!

Clinical Features

Taking Table 8.2 as a basic scheme, clinical features of fits and their equivalents in each age category will be considered in sequence.

Up to One Month

Up to the age of one month fits most frequently take the form of incomplete generalized convulsions with a tonic phase, and often apnoea, but no clonic phase. They may also be focal or multifocal, but a focal fit is less likely to

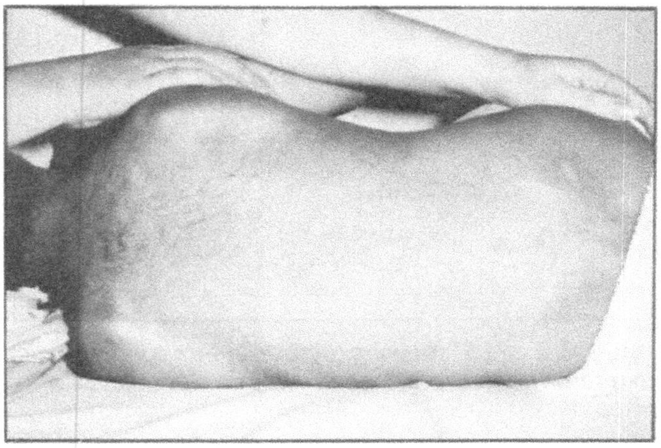

Figure 8.1. *Depigmented skin lesions, 'ash leaf spots', the only sign of tuberous sclerosis in a boy who presented with fits.*

indicate a localized neurological lesion than it is later in life. 'Jitteriness' in infants, a characteristic coarse tremor of the extremities at 10 cycles/second, may be mistaken for fitting but is generally benign. Apnoeic spells more frequently indicate serious disease and must be investigated whether or not they are due to fits.

Symptomatic Fits

During the neonatal period fits are almost invariably symptomatic, the most common causes being birth

Figure 8.2. *An infant with epilepsy and the Sturge-Weber syndrome, showing the typical capillary naevus involving the skin in the distribution of the ophthalmic branch of the trigeminal nerve.*

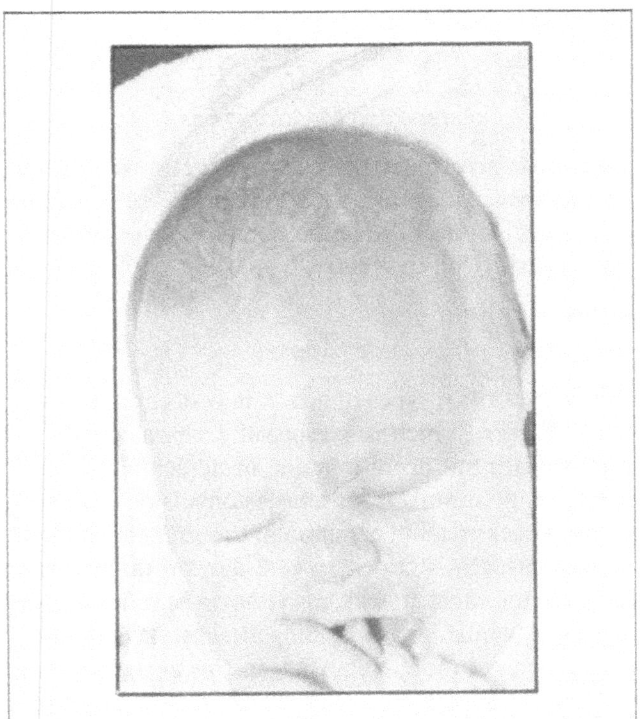

asphyxia, intracranial bleeding (especially in preterm infants) and metabolic disturbances such as hypocalcaemia and hypoglycaemia (especially in light-for-dates infants). Although fits are an unusual manifestation of neonatal meningitis this possibility must be excluded. It is apparent, therefore, that any newborn infant who has fits requires full investigation and close observation which is possible only in a properly staffed and equipped Special Care baby unit. The prognosis for neonatal fits depends on the underlying cause. Large intracranial (usually intraventricular) haemorrhages, meningitis and hypoglycaemia generally carry a grave prognosis, but the outlook otherwise is surprisingly hopeful and it is clear that fits in themselves are not damaging. For treatment we still prefer to use the well-tried anticonvulsants at this age, favouring paraldehyde for acute use and phenobarbitone for maintenance.

One Month to Six Months

Fits occur much less frequently during these months of life. The fully expressed grand mal convulsion remains unusual and, as in the younger infant, incomplete fits are more common. Infantile spasms may also start at this age; these are massive myoclonic spasms, usually flexor (hence another of the descriptive terms used for them, 'salaam spasms'), but occasionally extensor, which tend to occur in clusters with only a second or two between the brief spasms. This unusual fit pattern frequently goes unrecognized for some time and many infants are at first thought to have colic.

Breath-holding Attacks

Breath-holding attacks often start during these months although the peak age of onset is in the second half of the first year. They must be differentiated from fits. In a breath-holding attack an infant responds to a minor injury or frustration by starting to cry then fails to take another breath, nearly always in expiration and with mouth open, goes blue and limp and may show a few clonic twitches before breathing again and rapidly recovering. These attacks are entirely benign although terrifying for the onlookers. Some parents find they can prevent them by rapidly diverting the child's attention or curtail them by pulling the tongue forward or by mouth-to-mouth breathing. The most important therapeutic measures, however, are a full explanation and reassurance and the avoidance of anticonvulsants or sedatives, which are of no value.

Symptomatic Fits

In this age-group idiopathic fits remain very unusual. There is, therefore, a correspondingly high chance that fits will prove to be symptomatic and every effort must be made to elucidate the cause. Unfortunately, serious brain disease is frequently present, especially in children with the syndrome of infantile spasms. Approximately one third of these prove to have tuberous sclerosis, one third other serious brain disease and in one third the attacks remain unexplained. The EEG often shows a characteristic gross derangement known as 'hypsarrhythmia' (Figure 8.3). The fits may be difficult to control but valproate (Epilim), nitrazepam (Mogadon) and ACTH or prednisolone may prove effective. The fits tend to cease spontaneously after some months but these infants are often severely retarded.

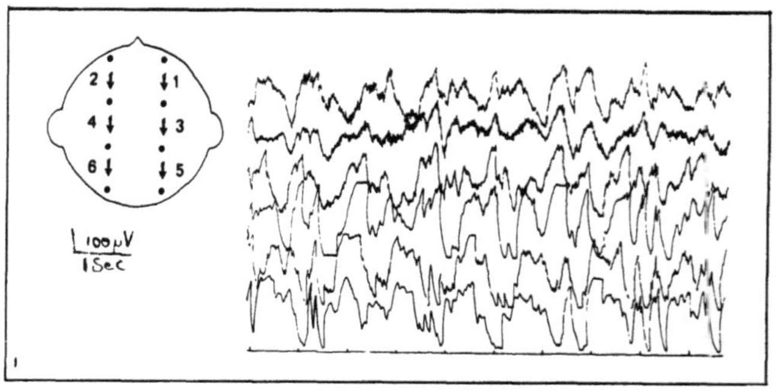

Figure 8.3. *EEG showing hypsarrhythmia, a chaotic mixture of generalized high amplitude slow waves and spikes.*

Six Months to Four Years

Febrile Convulsions

During this period of life the striking feature is the susceptibility of children to brief generalized fits provoked by fever. The tendency to febrile convulsions may be inherited and more than 90 per cent occur within this age range. As many as three to four per cent of all children have one febrile convulsion, but in only half this number are the attacks recurrent and only 10 to 15 per cent of this number continue to have fits after the third year of life. The source of the fever, as would be expected at this age, is most frequently a viral infection of the respiratory tract but the general practitioner's dilemma, seeing such a child at home, is to exclude more serious underlying infection, especially meningitis. It has been suggested that every child with a febrile convulsion should be referred to hospital but this is clearly impractical and, indeed, unnecessary, as it is often abundantly clear by the time the child is seen that no serious infection is present. Two important facts must be kept in mind: first, meningitis cannot be excluded reliably on clinical grounds before the age of two years, and second, many children with meningitis also have a red ear, a red throat or a 'rattly' chest. In order to avoid the dangers of inadequate or inappropriate treatment, it is therefore imperative that antibiotics are withheld until meningitis or other serious infection is excluded. When the general practitioner is in doubt, two courses are open to him: to refer the child to hospital immediately or to use symptomatic measures with control of the convulsion—cooling and antipyretics only—maintaining close observation until the situation is clarified. Although febrile convulsions are generally benign there is both experimental and clinical evidence to suggest that, if they are prolonged, cerebral anoxia may lead to damage in the temporal lobe causing a characteristic lesion (mesial horn sclerosis) which may later act as a focus for temporal lobe epilepsy. It is therefore a matter of urgency, as with all fits, to prevent a convulsion from becoming prolonged. This is usually best done with intravenous diazepam (Valium) or intramuscular paraldehyde. Intramuscular Valium is ineffective but it has recently been shown that the intravenous preparation is rapidly absorbed if instilled into the rectum. A 1 ml syringe can conveniently be used to instil half an ampoule (1 ml, 5 mg). This technique can be taught to parents of children with recurrent fits (Bower 1978).

The problem of prophylaxis for children with recurrent febrile convulsions is difficult. The convulsions can usually be prevented, but only by giving full doses of anticonvulsants for prolonged periods. Both phenobarbitone and valproate are effective (Wallace and Aldridge Smith, 1980). In the majority of children with febrile convulsions, however, long-term anticonvulsant therapy seems too high a price to pay for prophylaxis unless the fits are frequent, focal or prolonged beyond 15 minutes, start before the age of one year or occur in a child with a family history of febrile convulsions (*British Medical Journal* 1981).

Astatic and Myoclonic Fits

Astatic and myoclonic fits may also occur at this age and may escape diagnosis for a long time. These tend to occur in children with brain damage and control is frequently difficult to achieve.

Other Attacks

A number of other types of attack may occur in this age group. Rigors, which are especially characteristic of pyelonephritis but occur in many bacteraemic illnesses, are frequently mistaken for febrile convulsions. Breath-holding attacks remain common in the younger children but have usually stopped by the age of three years. Non-epileptic vagal attacks, also known as reflex anoxic seizures or 'white' breath-holding attacks, have recently been recognized more frequently in this age-group and are often misdiagnosed as fits. These attacks are probably due to vagally mediated reflex cardiac arrest and always follow some provocation, usually a minor injury. They can be differentiated from typical 'blue' breath-holding attacks by their more sudden onset, absence of a preliminary cry and pallor rather than cyanosis, but a brief anoxic seizure may frequently occur (Stephenson 1978). Anticonvulsants are ineffective but the attacks can be prevented by atropine. Masturbation in infants has occasionally led to a suspicion of epilepsy and anticonvulsant therapy is inappropriate!

Older than Four Years

Idiopathic Fits

The onset of idiopathic epilepsy generally occurs after the age of four years. The brain is now remarkably mature anatomically and, as in adults, although a wide variety of fits may occur, in the great majority of children these take highly stereotyped forms. Grand mal and temporal lobe fits are most common and are familiar to all doctors. Focal attacks occurring at this age usually indicate the presence of a focal neurological lesion. Petit mal is the most frequent form of minor epilepsy.

Cardiovascular Problems

A variety of conditions may mimic fits to a greater or lesser degree and many children have been, and no doubt currently are, maintained unnecessarily on anticonvulsants. It is increasingly appreciated that cardiovascular problems may be very misleading. The commonest and most familiar of these is, of course, the simple faint or vasovagal attack which is differentiated by the clear provocation, pallor, bradycardia and absence of ictal features. Unprovoked episodes of cardiac arrhythmia, such as those which occur with the 'sick sinus syndrome' and Wolff-Parkinson-White (Figure 8.4) conduction anomalies, may cause attacks which are more difficult to differentiate from fits. A high index of suspicion must be maintained and simple investigations should be made, such as the ECG, and followed up with prolonged rhythm recordings and other investigations if doubt persists. In congenital heart disease, Stokes-Adams attacks and cyanotic episodes may similarly resemble fits.

Other Attacks

Hysteria and simple malingering are rare in childhood and such attacks are generally bizarre enough to alert suspicion. In children with hypoglycaemia or hypocalcaemia, although the history or associated clinical findings may suggest the underlying metabolic problem, the attacks can be indistinguishable from idiopathic epilepsy, so these conditions must always be excluded chemically.

Epilepsy may be undiagnosed in the child, often brain-damaged, who shows wild outbursts and irrational behaviour. When these prove to be associated with fits, usually of temporal lobe origin, treatment with anticonvulsants may be extremely effective.

Narcolepsy, migraine, the periodic syndrome, night terrors, benign paroxysmal vertigo, drug-induced dyskinesias and no doubt many other conditions have caused confusion with epilepsy.

Figure 8.4. *The ECG of an eight-year-old boy who was observed by his medical father to have an episode of unconsciousness. Arrhythmia with an unstable pacemaker is present, some junctional beats and some complexes with features of the Wolff-Parkinson-White 'pre-excitation' conduction anomaly are shown. Further investigation confirmed episodes of arrhythmia.*

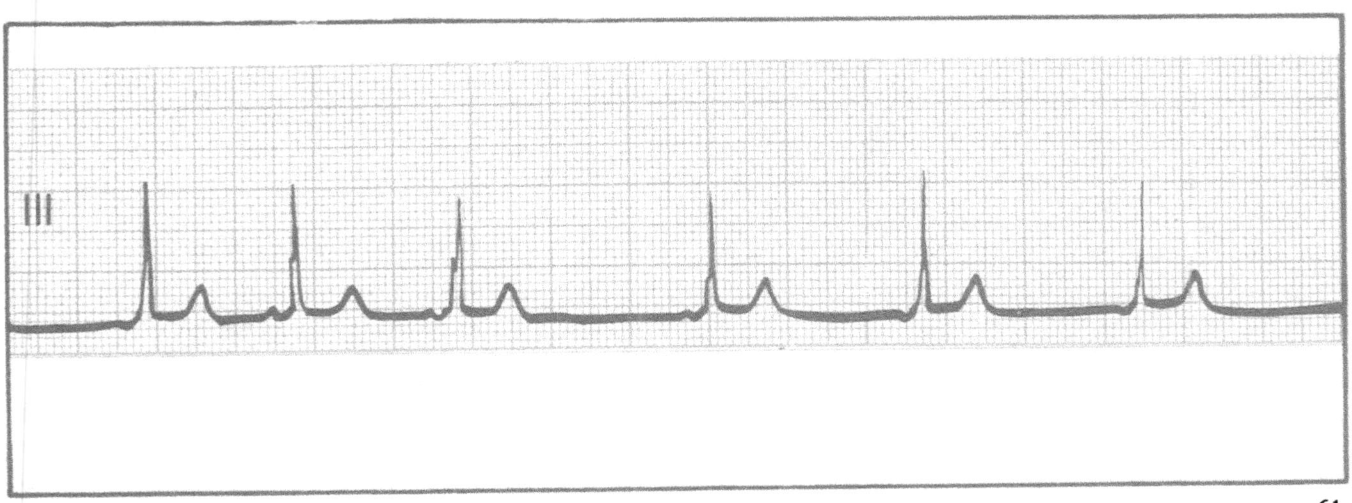

Investigation

In most children with recurrent fits an EEG and skull x-ray (Figure 8.5) are indicated and estimation of the fasting blood glucose and calcium is mandatory. The computerized tomographic scan has revolutionized the non-invasive investigation of the central nervous system and is the investigation of choice when a focal lesion is suspected (Figure 8.6). From the wide variety of conditions already considered it is apparent that, after preliminary screening tests, investigation may need to be pursued along one or more of many channels.

Treatment

Causes of symptomatic epilepsy must, as far as possible, be eradicated or treated. Idiopathic epilepsy can be fully controlled in the great majority of children. Some important facts about the major anticonvulsant drugs are summarized in Table 8.3. (See Figure 8.7.) Guiding principles in the drug treatment of epilepsy in childhood include:

1. The use of the least number of drugs (usually only one) with the least toxicity in the smallest effective dose.
2. The choice of as simple a dosage regime as possible. Children naturally dislike having to take tablets at school so a midday dose is likely to be 'forgotten'.
3. The use of blood anticonvulsant measurement for objective assessment of acceptance, dosage and absorption whenever problems arise.

Figure 8.5. *Skull radiograph of a nine-year-old girl who presented with fits and a facial haemangioma. Extensive linear ('tramline') calcification is shown, characteristic of the Sturge-Weber syndrome.*

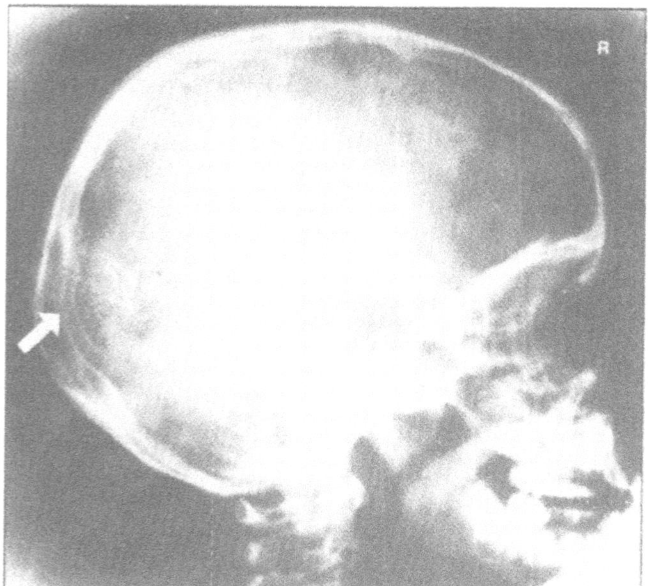

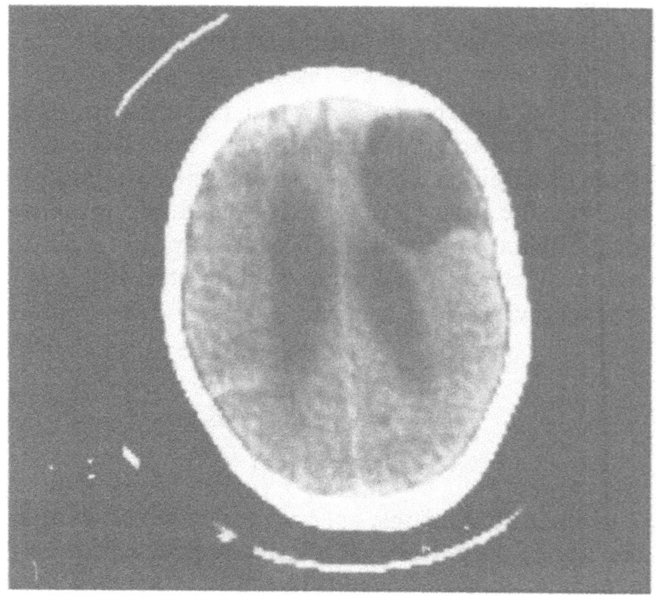

Figure 8.6. *A large porencephalic cyst demonstrated by CT scan in the right cerebral cortex of a child who presented with left-sided focal fits.*

4. Regular review of the continuing need for treatment. Many children can be weaned from treatment during childhood and it is our practice, unless there is a definite contraindication, to test the effect of a gradual reduction in the dose of an anticonvulsant in all children who have been free from fits for two years.

Valproate is the most recent important addition to the anticonvulsant armamentarium and has a chemical structure and mode of action entirely unlike the other major groups of compounds. It is proving a useful drug, especially in petit mal, and is well tolerated by children and generally free from side-effects. Unfortunately, fatal liver toxicity has recently been reported in several cases, and it is therefore recommended that liver function tests are checked regularly. A moderate rise in serum enzyme levels is frequently seen and the drug should be stopped if this exceeds three times the normal value, or any other abnormality is observed. It is not clear whether this precaution will prove sufficient to anticipate the exceptional severe idiosyncratic response (Browne 1980).

Problems in Management

Finally, some of the many problems which arise in the management of epilepsy in childhood will be considered:

Status epilepticus, in which there is continuous or sequential fitting without recovery of consciousness for more than 30 minutes, is a serious medical emergency

Table 8.3. Major anticonvulsant drugs used in children.

Drug	Indications	Route	Dose	Problems
Diazepam (Valium)	Acute use in prolonged or recurrent fits	a) slow i.v. b) rectal	0.2-0.3 mg/kg 5 mg	Respiratory depression
Paraldehyde	Acute use in prolonged or recurrent fits	Deep i.m.	0.15 ml/kg, or 1 ml/year of age	Local tissue damage
Carbamazepine (Tegretol)	Grand mal Temporal lobe Focal	Oral	Up to 20 mg/kg in two doses	Transient fatigue, irritability, ataxia, rash. Very rarely serious blood toxicity
Phenytoin (Epanutin)	Grand mal Temporal lobe Other focal	Oral	4-6 mg/kg in one or two doses	Variable pharmacokinetics, blood levels especially important Toxicity: acute—ataxia, nystagmus; chronic—hirsutism (Figure 8.7), gum hypertrophy, facial coarsening, behaviour disturbance, rarely serious blood disorders, rickets, lupus and other 'allergic' problems
Valproate (Epilim)	Petit mal, atypical petit mal Myoclonic Grand mal Prophylaxis of febrile convulsions	Oral	20-50 mg/kg in two or three doses	Short plasma half-life but b.d. dosage often effective. Transient GI upsets, drowsiness, hair loss, increased serum hepatic enzyme levels, rarely thrombocytopenia, severe liver toxicity, pancreatitis
Phenobarbitone	Newborn Prophylaxis of febrile convulsions	Oral	4-6 mg/kg in one or two doses	Very common adverse effects on mood, learning and behaviour

more common in the younger age-groups. Any child who fails to respond to treatment with intravenous or rectal diazepam or intramuscular paraldehyde (Table 8.3) within a few minutes should be transferred as rapidly as possible to hospital.

Inadequate control of fits may be due to misdiagnosis, intercurrent illness, failure to take the drugs prescribed, inadequate dosage or use of the wrong drugs and all these must be excluded before the fit is ascribed to intractable epilepsy. Sorting out these possibilities may require much clinical skill.

Psychological, emotional and educational problems. Epilepsy is a condition which for many people still carries overtones of devilish possession and the supernatural. The child and his relatives are likely, therefore, to harbour all sorts of extraordinary and irrational anxieties which can be removed only by full discussion and reassurance. The epileptic child is also likely to feel different and set apart from his peers by his illness. In spite of this, we feel strongly that it is desirable for epileptic children to attend normal schools whenever possible. On the other hand, some contact with other parents and children with the same problem is often

Figure 8.7. *Phenytoin-induced hirsutism in an epileptic girl.*

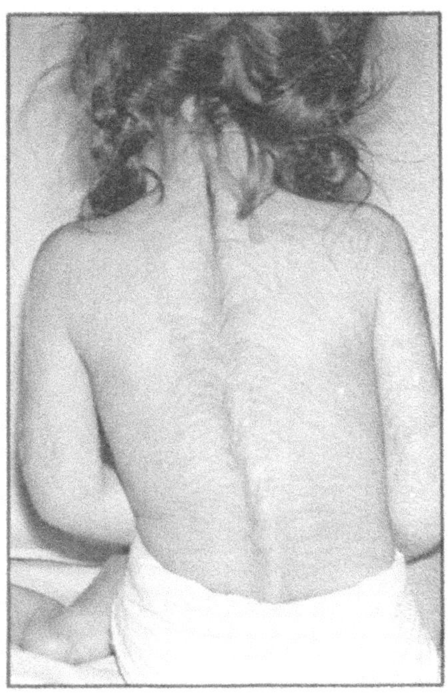

helpful. To some extent this is achieved in a specialized hospital clinic but lay societies, such as the British Epilepsy Association, can provide help in many dimensions the best doctor cannot reach, so even non-joiners should be encouraged to sample them. The epileptic child who is under-achieving intellectually, socially or athletically presents another complex but intriguing conundrum. Is the problem due to the fits themselves, underlying brain disease, the drugs or emotional disturbance? The general practitioner is often in the best position to decide and to help.

Limitations on activity. Most children greatly resent restrictions, and indeed some reject them outright, thus exposing themselves to dangers they might otherwise have avoided. It is, therefore, both sensible and prudent to impose only limitations which seem absolutely essential and reasonably practicable even when this involves an element of physical risk.

Fears for the future. Parents and children are grateful for early discussion and advice on such matters as driving licences, career choices, marriage and the prognosis of offspring.

Fortunately the problem of epilepsy in childhood seldom proves to be as bad as it first appears either to the child or his relatives, so the well-informed, optimistic and supportive family doctor has a unique opportunity to alleviate the burden of this feared disease.

References

Bower, B., *Br. J. Hosp. Med.*, 1978, **19**, 8.

British Medical Journal (editorial), 1981, **282**, 673.

Browne, T. R., *New Engl. J. Med.*, 1980, **302**, 661.

Ross, E. M., Peckham, C. S., West, P. B. and Butler, N. R., *Br. Med. J.*, 1980, **280**, 207.

Stephenson, J. B. P., *Arch. Dis. Childh.*, 1978, **53**, 193.

Wallace, S. J. and Aldridge Smith, J., *Br. Med. J.*, 1980, **280**, 353.

Further Reading

Wallace, S. J., in *Paediatric Neurology*, Ed. F. C. Rose, Blackwell Scientific Publications, Oxford, 1979, p. 346.

9. Congenital Heart Disease

A sense of insecurity is commonly experienced by the doctor assessing a child with suspected congenital heart disease (CHD). Such anxiety is unnecessary. Although the subject is one of great complexity for the paediatric cardiologist and cardiac surgeon, the rules for safe practice in primary care are straightforward and the knowledge and skills required for a competent first assessment by no means overwhelming.

Loud warning bells should be sounded by cardiac cyanosis, heart failure and findings indicating tight outflow tract obstruction. These are indications to seek expert assistance without delay. The rare but ever-present danger of bacterial endocarditis must not be forgotten; the parents of children with CHD should be given an instruction sheet such as that shown in Table 9.1. With these simple principles in mind, a contemplative rather than an aggressive approach to the problem can be safely adopted!

Incidence

Six children in 1,000 are born with structural heart disease. The relative incidence of the more common defects in children surviving infancy is shown in Figure 9.1. It is apparent that, of more than 100 recognized lesions, only eight are at all common and they account

Figure 9.1. *Relative incidence of common congenital heart defects in children after infancy.*

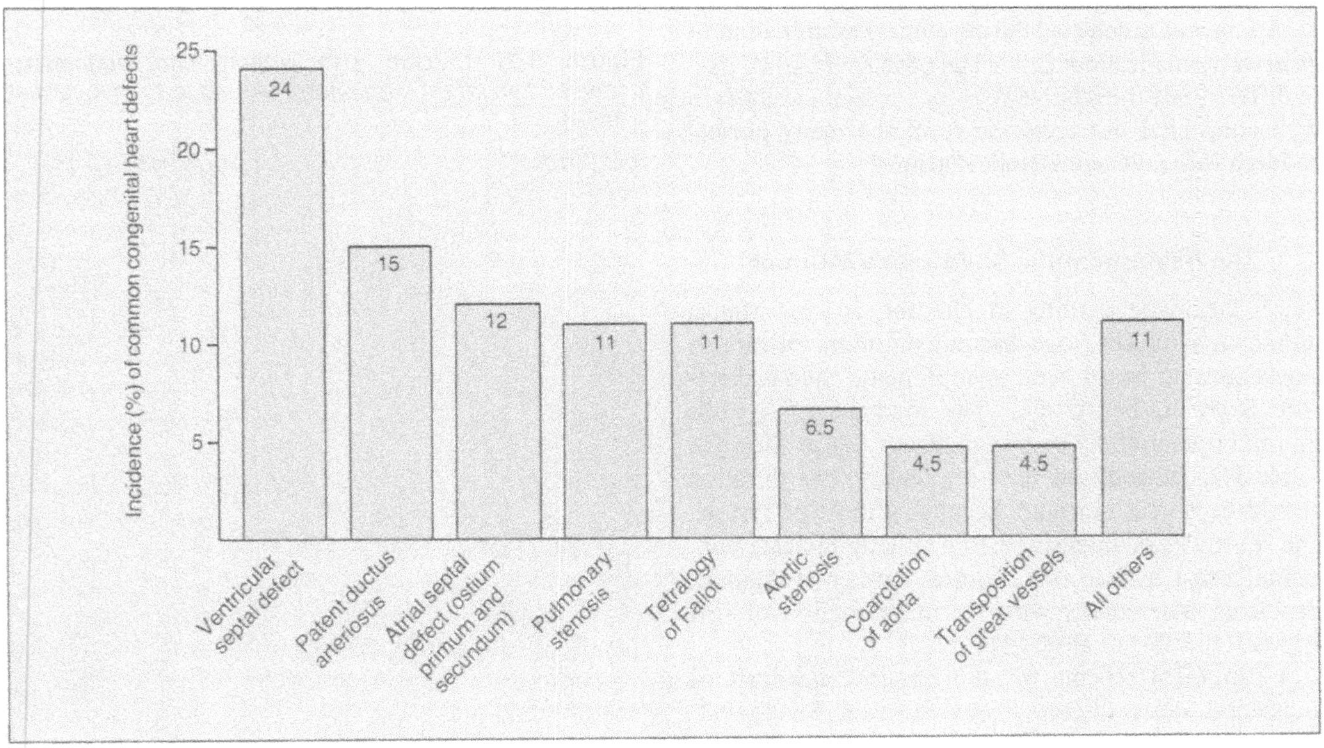

for nearly 90 per cent of all CHD. Of these, only two are cyanotic, Fallot's tetralogy and transposition of the great vessels; the rest involve either a left to right shunt or an obstructive lesion.

Presentation

Some severe forms of CHD are incompatible with extrauterine life; about 10 per cent of affected infants die within the neonatal period and contribute about 10 per cent of all neonatal deaths. The others nearly all present in one of three ways:

1. A systolic murmur is heard in the first few days of life. The majority of these babies do not have CHD: the murmur is due to turbulent blood flow associated with the high neonatal cardiac output (250 ml/kg/min. from each ventricle) and the change from the fetal to the adult circulatory pattern. If the infant is asymptomatic, the best course is masterly inactivity in the hope that the murmur will go away. If in seven to ten days it has not done so, the infant should be reassessed.

2. The child develops symptoms or signs of cyanosis or heart failure. In infancy, heart failure causes failure to thrive, feeding difficulty, tachypnoea and breathlessness, cough and enlargement of the liver. Oedema is unusual. The chest x-ray shows cardiac enlargement (Figure 9.2). The child with CHD who develops heart failure usually does so within the first few months of life. In older children heart failure is rare, and the signs and symptoms are those found in adults. Children with cyanosis or heart failure should be referred to a specialized cardiac unit without delay.

3. A murmur is detected during clinical examination of an asymptomatic older child. The problem is, of course, to differentiate the relatively few asymptomatic children with congenital heart disease from the many normal children with innocent systolic murmurs.

The Asymptomatic Child with a Murmur

Since rheumatic carditis in children is now almost unknown in the UK, lone diastolic murmurs are rare. A single murmur heard in an asymptomatic child is therefore likely to be systolic. The loudness of systolic murmurs can usefully be graded from 1 to 6 as shown in Table 9.2. In addition to the intensity, the duration should be noted: murmurs occupying most of systole, and murmurs of intensity 3 to 6 usually indicate congenital heart disease that requires further evaluation. Problems arise chiefly with the interpretation of soft systolic murmurs of grades 1 and 2.

A simplified scheme for the physical diagnosis of congenital heart disease is presented in Figure 9.3. Having excluded cyanosis and heart failure, the next

Table 9.1. Instruction sheet for parents of children with congenital heart disease.

Antibiotic prophylaxis for children with congenital heart disease

Children with congenital heart disease are at risk from bacterial endocarditis. Good care of the teeth is essential. Any dental procedure likely to cause bleeding may release bacteria into the circulation. A prophylactic antibiotic should therefore be given. Suitable regimes (half doses for children under 8 years) are:

Intramuscular penicillin, given 1 hour before the procedure

Triplopen 1 vial i.m. is a convenient sustained-action preparation

If penicillin G is given continue with oral penicillin as below for 48 hours

Oral penicillin V, 500 mg 1 hour before procedure then 250 mg 6 hourly for 48 hours

For children sensitive to penicillin:

Oral erythromycin, 500 mg 1 hour before procedure then 250 mg 6 hourly for 48 hours

(Suitable antibiotic cover is necessary for procedures on the upper respiratory tract, gastrointestinal tract and genito-urinary tract)

Please show this sheet to your child's dentist before any procedure is carried out

Figure 9.2. *Cardiac enlargement and pulmonary oedema in an infant with heart failure due to myocardial disease.*

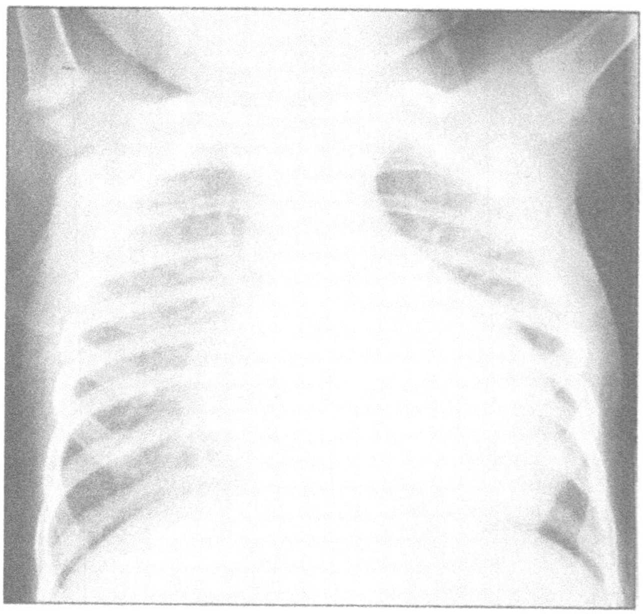

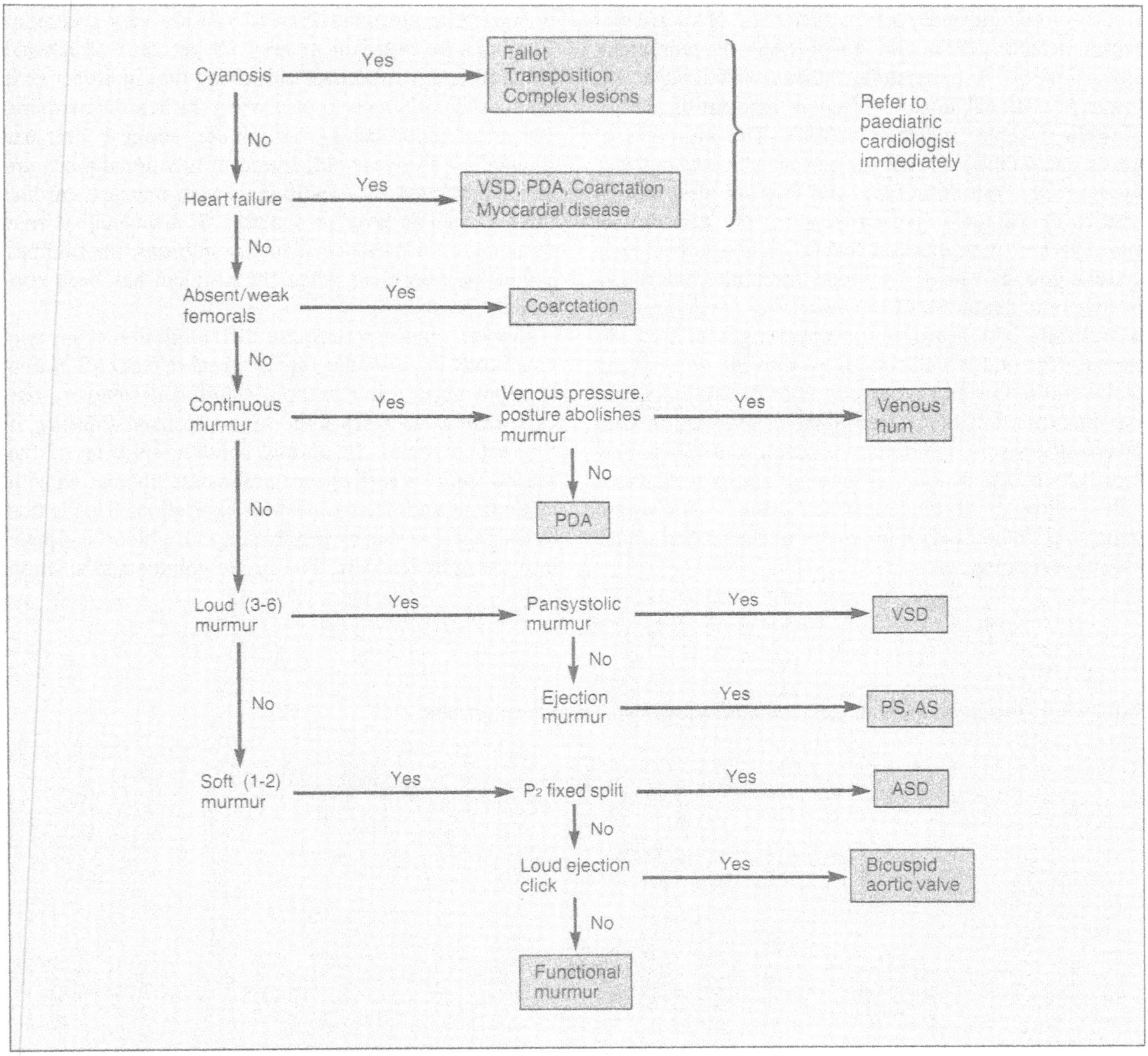

Figure 9.3. *A simplified scheme for the physical diagnosis of congenital heart disease.*

step is to feel the femoral pulses. If these are absent, or weak in comparison with the brachials, the diagnosis is coarctation of the aorta. Next, the murmur is evaluated.

Continuous Murmurs

A continuous murmur, apparently spilling over from systole through all or most of diastole, is likely to be due to a venous hum or a patent ductus. A venous hum can usually be abolished by turning the head to one side or by occluding the veins at the base of the neck. The classical 'machinery' murmur of patent ductus, of maximal intensity under the left clavicle, generally extends well into diastole except in infants in the first few months of life. Prominent peripheral pulses and a wide pulse pressure are further clues to a patent ductus.

Table 9.2. Grading of heart murmurs according to loudness.

Grade	Loudness on auscultation
1	Soft, just audible
2	Easily heard
3	Loud and clear without thrill
4	Loud and clear with thrill
5	Between 4 and 6!
6	Heard without stethoscope

Loud Systolic Murmurs

Loud systolic murmurs are characteristic of ventricular septal defects (VSD) and aortic (AS) or pulmonary stenosis (PS). A pansystolic murmur maximal at the lower left sternal border, often in association with a diastolic rumble, indicates a VSD. The murmurs of aortic and pulmonary stenosis may also be long but they are typically ejection in type, and they are often associated with palpable hypertrophy of the appropriate ventricle and with ejection 'clicks', high-pitched early systolic sounds caused by blood forcefully entering a poststenotic dilatation of the vessel. An aortic murmur is generally best heard at the upper right or mid left sternal edge and is well conducted into the neck. Weak peripheral pulses and a narrow pulse pressure confirm the diagnosis but are present only in association with severe stenosis. A pulmonary ejection murmur is best heard at the upper left sternal edge and is well transmitted through to the upper left back. With severe stenosis the pulmonary component of the second sound may be soft or inaudible.

Soft Systolic Murmurs

Soft systolic murmurs (Figure 9.4) are very common. They can be heard in at least 20 per cent of normal children and it is perhaps surprising that in 80 per cent no audible turbulence occurs when the heart is pumping 100 ml of blood per kg per minute, about 2 litres per minute in a five-year-old! Innocent functional murmurs are accentuated by conditions which increase cardiac output, such as fever or anaemia. If a murmur is first detected in the presence of such conditions, the findings should be reassessed when the problem has been corrected.

Innocent murmurs require differentiation from two conditions in particular, atrial septal defect (ASD) and bicuspid aortic valve without significant stenosis. The chief clue to an ASD is the wide and fixed splitting of the second sound. In normal children splitting of the second sound is easily heard at the base, increasing with inspiration and decreasing with expiration. This is due to the fact that during inspiration more blood is drawn into the right ventricle. The stroke volume and ejection

Figure 9.4. *Auscultation findings in conditions with soft systolic murmurs.*

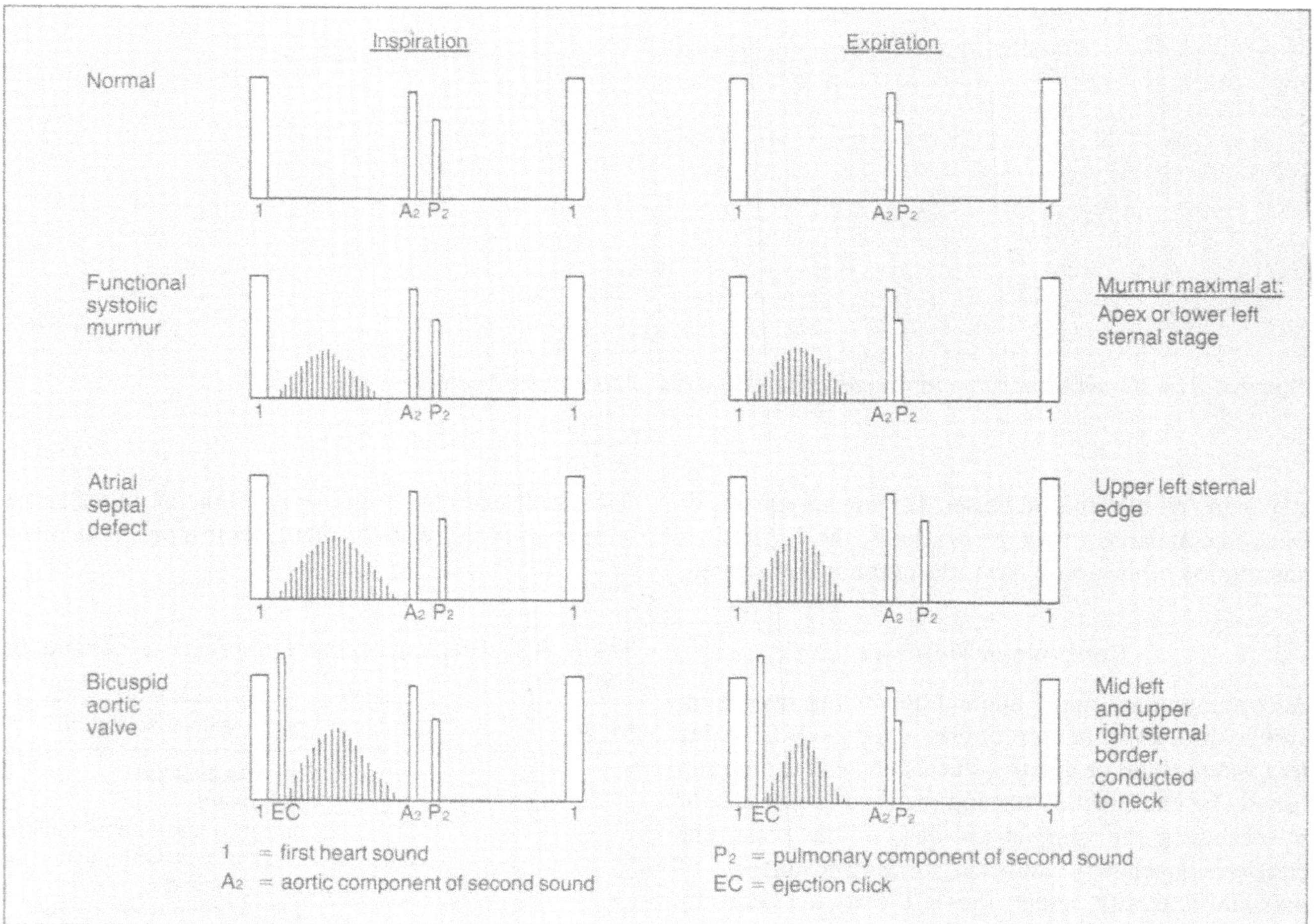

time of the ventricle increase accordingly and the pulmonary valve closes later in relation to the aortic valve. In the presence of an ASD, however, there is free communication between the atria and ventricular filling is determined by the relative compliance of the two ventricles. This results in wide splitting of the second sound which does not alter with the phase of inspiration.

It is fortunately not a matter of tremendous moment if an ASD is missed or the murmur mistaken for an innocent murmur; ASD is usually asymptomatic until adult life and bacterial endocarditis almost never occurs. A lesion of greater importance is the bicuspid aortic valve. If this is not associated with significant stenosis the systolic murmur may be very soft or absent. The characteristic physical sign is a loud aortic ejection click. Bacterial endocarditis may occur on a bicuspid valve and can rapidly produce serious aortic incompetence; calcific aortic stenosis may occur in bicuspid valves in later life.

The functional nature of a systolic murmur may be surmised when none of these features is present. In addition, innocent murmurs are generally accentuated when the child is lying flat, they are often 'musical' in quality and heard maximally at the left sternal edge and are not conducted widely.

Conclusion

Thus clues to the diagnosis of all the common forms of congenital heart disease can be gleaned from careful physical examination with attention especially to the peripheral pulses, murmurs and the second heart sound. In the absence of such clues a confident diagnosis of innocence can be made. QED!

Further Reading

Scott, O. and Jordan, S. C., *Heart Disease in Paediatrics,* Butterworth, London, 1973.

10. Renal Tract Problems

DISEASE of the renal tract in childhood, as in adult life, is frequently silent. It is therefore necessary to maintain continuous vigilance and a high degree of diagnostic suspicion. It is a sad experience to see a child present for the first time with growth failure or hypertensive encephalopathy due to advanced renal failure when the history reveals that warning signs of underlying renal disease have been underestimated or ignored in the past. Urine testing is the cornerstone of diagnosis and, for the patient, is the simplest of all investigations. There can be no compromise on the absolute rule that every ill child in whom full and sufficient cause is not apparent *must* have urine analysis.

Urinary Tract Infection (UTI)

It has been estimated that at least five per cent of girls will have a UTI before they leave school. In boys, the incidence is probably less than one per cent (Smellie and Normand 1976). The recognition of UTI is important not only for the prevention and treatment of acute symptoms, but also for the prevention of renal damage which may lead to renal failure.

Symptoms

The symptoms of UTI range from none at all to the full syndrome of pyelonephritis with fever, rigors, loin pain, dysuria, frequency and haematuria. It is important to emphasize that UTI symptoms in children are often different from those in adults.

UTI in Neonates

UTI in the first two weeks of life usually presents with mild and nonspecific symptoms. It occurs in 0.5 to 1.0 per cent of all babies. Any infant showing one or more of the following symptoms or signs must have urine analysis:

1. Either a mild increase in body temperature or hypothermia.
2. Poor weight gain.
3. Poor feeding with or without vomiting and diarrhoea.
4. General listlessness and malaise.
5. Persisting jaundice.

UTI in Infancy

Patients under 18 months of age are obviously unable to complain of dysuria, and frequency is concealed by the nappies. A UTI should be suspected in an infant with:

1. Fever, for which no obvious reason can be found.
2. Prolonged anaemia, particularly if it does not respond to iron therapy.
3. Jaundice, especially in the first two months of life.
4. Failure to thrive, or other nonspecific illness.

UTI in Older Children

In this age-group, children frequently present with fever, vomiting and abdominal pain or with symptoms more similar to those which occur in adults. Haematuria is found in only about 10 per cent of children with urinary tract infection. One important symptom of infection in childhood is secondary enuresis, i.e. enuresis starting after at least a six-month period of night-time dryness.

Signs

The signs of UTI are also vague and nonspecific. Flank tenderness may be detected at any age by gentle palpation in the renal angles. If pyelonephritis is present and the kidneys are tender this will make the child wince or cry. Suprapubic tenderness is not generally a helpful sign. A urine sample must be examined if any urinary tract symptoms are present irrespective of positive physical findings in other systems.

Differential Diagnosis

The most important differential diagnosis is local infection—balanitis in boys and vulvovaginitis in girls. The latter, especially, may mimic a UTI with frequency and dysuria, though systemic symptoms are usually absent. This symptom complex is very common. Urine collected through the topically infected genitalia may then 'confirm' a spurious diagnosis of UTI. It is essential to examine the genitalia of children of either sex with urinary symptoms.

Diagnosis

The criteria for the diagnosis of UTI are clear, and are summarized in Table 10.1. If these criteria are not met, the diagnosis of UTI is not proven.

It is important that reports such as those shown in Table 10.2 are not considered diagnostic of UTI—particularly in girls who may have had vulvovaginitis, or in whom collection of a satisfactory urine sample may have proved difficult.

Table 10.1. Diagnostic criteria for urinary tract infections.

1. In a freshly voided unspun specimen more than 20 white cells per mm^3 in boys, or more than 50 white cells per mm^3 in girls, *and*
More than 10^5 organisms per ml in pure culture.

2. In a suprapubic puncture specimen more than 10^3 organisms per ml and any WBC.

Table 10.2. Typical MSU results which are insufficient to sustain a diagnosis of UTI.

1. WBC	20/mm^3
E. coli	10^4/ml
Strep. faecalis	10^4/ml
2. WBC	50/mm^3
E. coli	10^4/ml
Proteus	10^3/ml
3. WBC	5/mm^3
E. coli	10^4–10^5/ml
4. WBC	200/mm^3
Staph. aureus	10^4/ml
5. WBC	More than 5/mm^3
E. coli	10^5/ml
Strep. faecalis	10^5/ml

In cases where the urine has been collected in a urine bag, the results must also be viewed with grave suspicion because contamination occurs so readily. If the urine is clear, the child certainly does not have a UTI. Only a really impressive result, e.g. more than 200 WBC per mm^3, and a pure growth of more than 10^5/ml *E. coli* in the absence of genital infection, can be considered proof of infection.

Another report that should engender suspicion in a first UTI is growth of an organism other than *E. coli* or, in boys, *Proteus.*

The general practitioner may protest that such counsels of perfection are applicable only to the hospital-based paediatrician with good laboratory back-up. However, since *all* children with UTI require x-rays of their renal tract, it is crucially important to establish whether UTI is present or not.

The general practitioner confronted with a symptomatic patient demanding immediate therapy should note the following relevant points:

1. Cloudy urine alone does *not* indicate UTI.
2. Albuminuria alone does *not* indicate UTI.
3. The uricult method is a satisfactory technique for obtaining a semiquantitative urinary culture.
4. The only reliable quick test, and the one we use in the children's wards, casualty and outpatient departments, is microscopy of the fresh urine. Pyuria greater than 50 WBC/mm^3 in the absence of topical infection indicates UTI.

The organisms usually cultured in UTIs are listed in Table 10.3. The figure of two per cent for initial infections due to *Proteus* is probably low in view of recent studies which have suggested that as many as 25 per cent of initial UTIs in boys are due to that organism.

Investigation

Once UTI has been confirmed, an intravenous urogram (IVU) must be carried out in all children. It is our practice to obtain a micturating cystourethrogram as well in children up to five years of age. Approximately

Table 10.3. Infecting organisms in urinary tract infection.

Organism	Primary infection (%)	Recurrent infection (%)
E. coli	91	59
Proteus	2	20
Enterococci	4	6
Others	3	15

25 per cent of children show a radiological abnormality, most commonly ureteric reflux with or without pyelonephritic scarring of the kidneys. Some of the abnormalities which may be found are illustrated in Figures 10.1, 10.2, 10.3, 10.4, and 12.5 (page 88).

The presence of reflux is crucial in the development of pyelonephritic scarring, although it remains to be determined whether reflux on its own, or reflux plus intrarenal reflux (reflux into the tubules themselves), or reflux plus infection is required for renal parenchymal damage to occur. Fortunately, it is rare for new scarring to develop after the age of five years. Indeed, increasingly strong evidence suggests that reflux, if it is going to cause kidney scarring, does so either in utero or early in infancy. Hence the importance of carrying out micturating cystourethrography in all infants with a first UTI, and recognizing UTI as quickly as possible in infants and toddlers. It seems reasonable to omit micturating cystourethrography in children over five years of age with normal IVU.

We do not routinely investigate renal function, even with simple tests such as urea and electrolytes, unless the radiographs show some abnormality.

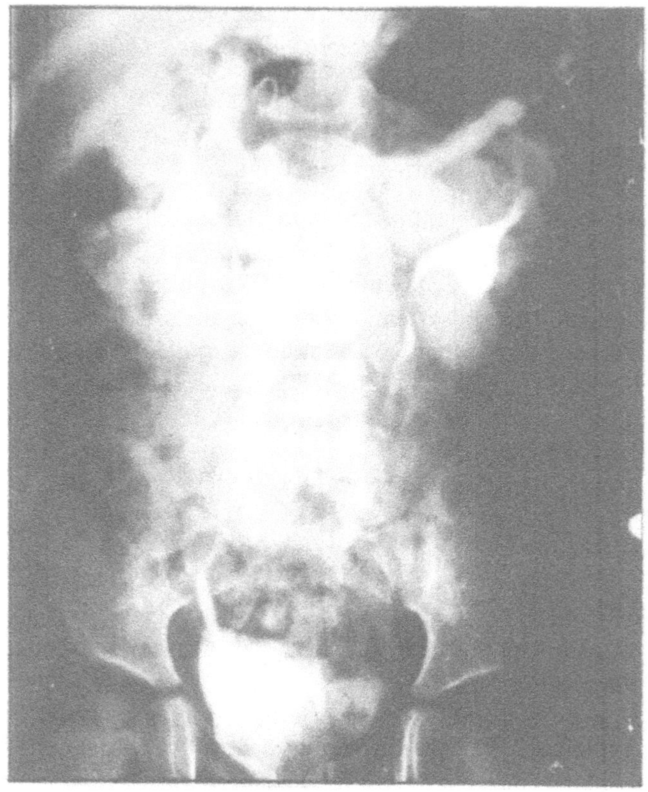

Figure 10.2. *Ectopic ureterocele. The IVU shows no contrast in the left upper pelvis, which is drained by the non-functioning ureter, and a filling defect in the bladder where the ectopic ureter opens into the urethra and forms a ureterocele.*

Treatment

The standard treatment for UTI is a one-week course of co-trimoxazole, a sulphonamide or trimethoprim. Other agents should be used only if there is a history of drug hypersensitivity or when indicated by appropriate bacterial sensitivity tests.

If the radiological assessment shows a minor degree of ureteric reflux, long-term treatment with low-dose (one-half to one-third normal dose) treatment is indicated. The renal tract radiology should be checked every 18 to 24 months, and the co-trimoxazole, nitrofurantoin or trimethoprim continued until reflux has resolved. If reflux is severe, if renal scarring is present or if it proves difficult to control infection medically, then surgical reimplantation of the refluxing ureters should be considered but the indications for this operation remain controversial.

Figure 10.1. *The IVU showing bilateral calyceal deformities and cortical scarring in a 12-year-old girl with chronic pyelonephritis.*

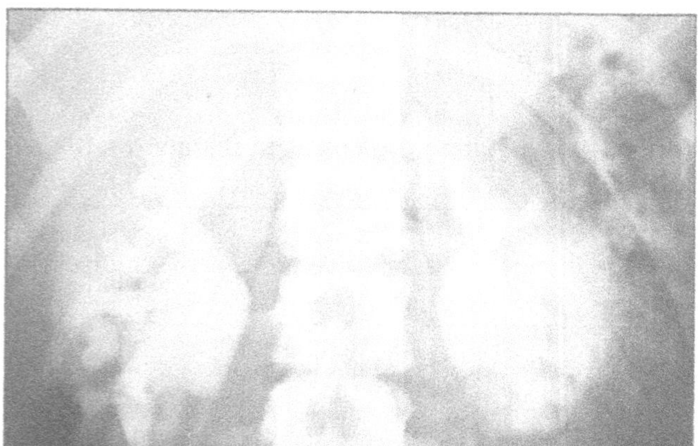

Three other aspects of treatment are important. A liberal fluid intake lowers the osmolality of the renal medulla and helps to eliminate L forms of bacteria lodging there. Double micturition should be practised to ensure that urine refluxing up the ureter during the initial micturition is emptied out completely, thereby preventing urinary stasis which encourages infection. Finally, constipation predisposes to UTI so a regular bowel action shoud be ensured.

Follow-up

After a course of treatment, urinalysis to check that the infection has been eradicated is, of course, mandatory. Thereafter, three-monthly urinalysis should ideally be continued for at least one year. Children on long-term antibiotics should also have their urine checked at least three-monthly during treatment and for one year afterwards.

Asymptomatic Bacteriuria

Population surveys show that between 1.5 and 2.0 per cent of girls have asymptomatic bacteriuria, which can be diagnosed only when two successive urine specimens show a pure growth of more than 10^5 organisms/ml. Strictly speaking, the bacteriuria may not be entirely asymptomatic, since many of these girls have some slight frequency, enuresis or daytime wetting. In spite of the mild symptoms, they should have the same radiological investigations as children with symptomatic UTI because they show a similar incidence of anatomical abnormality. The correct treatment for such children is uncertain. In those without radiological abnormality there is probably little point in using antibiotics, since the infection frequently recurs when they are withdrawn. In those children with radiological abnormality, it seems wise to use treatment similar to that for symptomatic UTI.

The Child with Persistent Relapsing UTI and Normal Radiographs

Such children are not uncommon. Faulty vulval hygiene, incomplete emptying of the bladder and constipation may be factors predisposing to infection. Girls should be advised to bath frequently but not to add

Figure 10.3. *Megaureter-megacystis. The cystogram shows gross dilatation of the collecting system in a child with a severely dysplastic renal tract.*

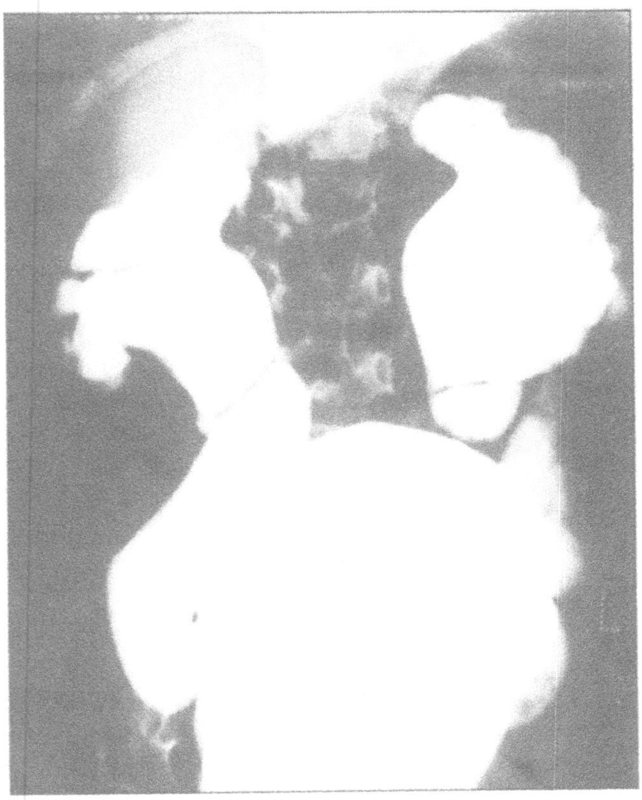

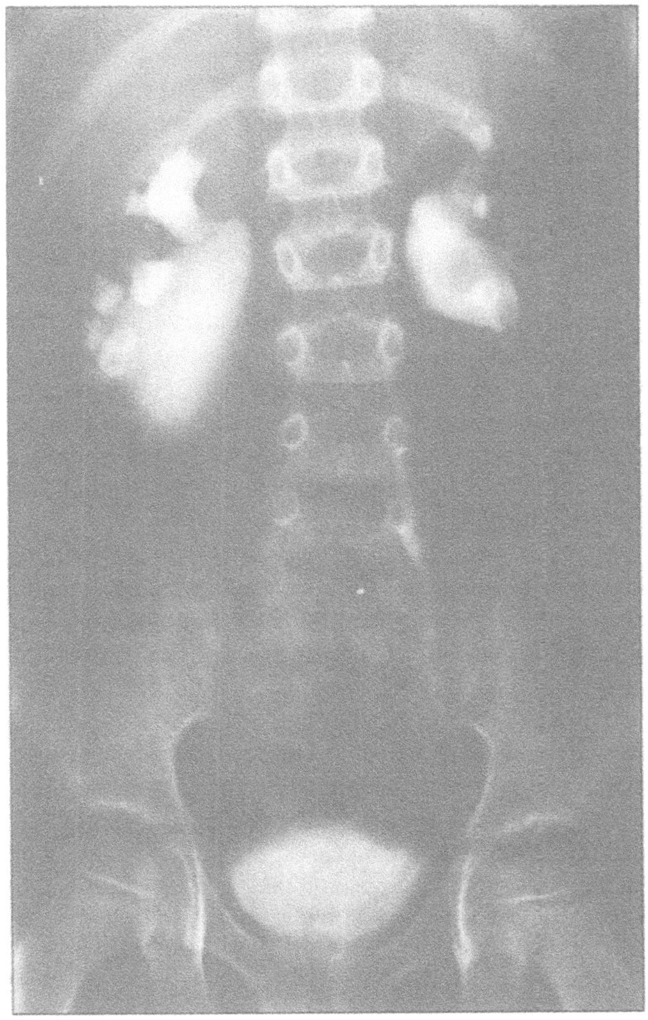

Figure 10.4. *Bilateral pelviureteric obstruction in a nine-year-old boy who presented with recurrent urinary tract infection.*

disinfectants, detergents or commercial bath additives to the bath water. They should not use underwear made from synthetic fibres and should avoid contamination of the introitus after defaecation. They should drink plenty of fluids, practise double micturition and avoid constipation. If necessary, a prolonged course of low-dose prophylactic treatment (as above) will prevent reinfection and the recurrence of unpleasant symptoms. Dilatation of the urethra under general anaesthesia may occasionally be helpful in girls.

Enuresis

Enuresis is one of the commonest problems in medical paediatrics. At least 10 per cent of children still wet the bed at night at the age of five years. In the majority, enuresis represents a phenomenon of maturational delay and 15 to 20 per cent of these children achieve nocturnal continence during each subsequent year.

Secondary enuresis is much less common. In some children it simply represents a temporary loss of control, in others it is a manifestation of emotional stress, and, most important, it may be the presenting sign of a UTI or other organic problem.

When assessing primary enuresis it is important to ascertain that urinary control during the day is normal. Abnormalities of the genitalia or lumbosacral spine (Figures 10.5, 10.6 and 10.7) must be sought on examination. In both primary and secondary enuresis it is also important to exclude urinary infection. In younger children, overt stress is rarely a cause of enuresis and psychiatric evaluation is seldom indicated. In older children, particularly those with secondary enuresis, psychiatric factors may be crucial, and cure of the enuresis dependent upon their solution.

In primary enuresis, or secondary enuresis without infection or major psychiatric factors, the treatment most likely to prove successful is the combination of an enuretic alarm buzzer and a tricyclic antidepressant drug, such as imipramine or amitriptyline. It is not clear whether these drugs work centrally or peripherally but they are frequently effective. In overdose they are also extremely dangerous so it must be strongly emphasized to the parents that the drug must be kept in a locked and entirely childproof medicine cabinet. When the alarm buzzer is used it is important that it is used correctly. The child must wake when the buzzer sounds (which may require a loud buzzer, drugs to lighten sleep or employment of a parent to wake the child when the alarm goes off), he must get up, turn off the buzzer and then go to empty his bladder. If this routine is followed regularly, from 80 to 90 per cent of enuretics will become dry within two months.

Figure 10.5. *A large lumbosacral meningomyelocele after operative closure. Wasting of the limbs and a healed bedsore are also visible.*

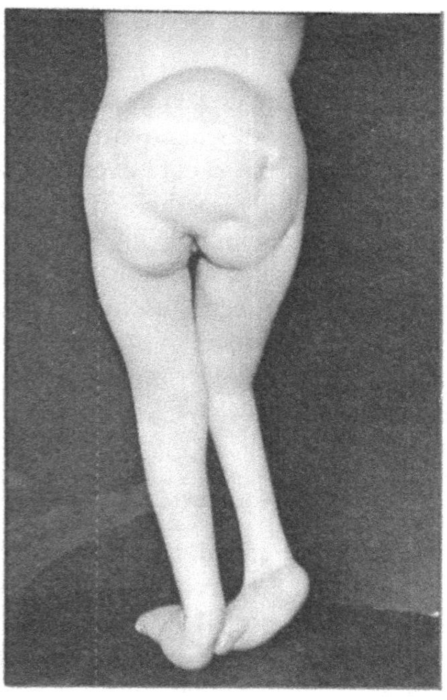

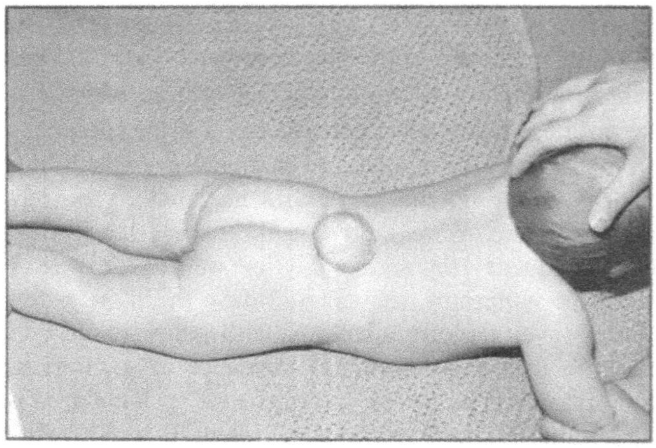

Figure 10.6. *An unoperated lumbar meningocele.*

Haematuria

It is traditional to introduce this topic by reminding readers that all red urine is not haematuria. The differential diagnosis of true haematuria is given in Table 10.4. Clearly, we cannot discuss all these conditions individually. Haematuria should always be investigated and the tests which should be carried out routinely, and in other special circumstances, are outlined in Table 10.5. The problem was well reviewed by West (1976). Often the cause is obvious, for instance, with a history of trauma, local evidence of meatal ulcer or perineal soreness, stigmata of specific illness such as haemolytic uraemic syndrome, Henoch-Schönlein purpura (Figure 10.8) or septicaemia, or symptoms of urinary tract infection or renal calculus. Although urinary tract infection is an important cause of haematuria in childhood, only 10 per cent of children with UTI show haematuria. In children with painless haematuria, an IVU should be carried out to exclude neoplasm and to delineate any renal malformation, such as polycystic kidneys. This leaves the various nephritides for further discussion.

Acute Glomerulonephritis

Whether because of the secular trend towards better general health, altered virulence of the Group A beta haemolytic streptococcus, or the widespread use of antibiotics to treat streptococcal throat infections, acute glomerulonephritis is now a rare disease in the UK. The classical pentad of findings, preceding streptococcal

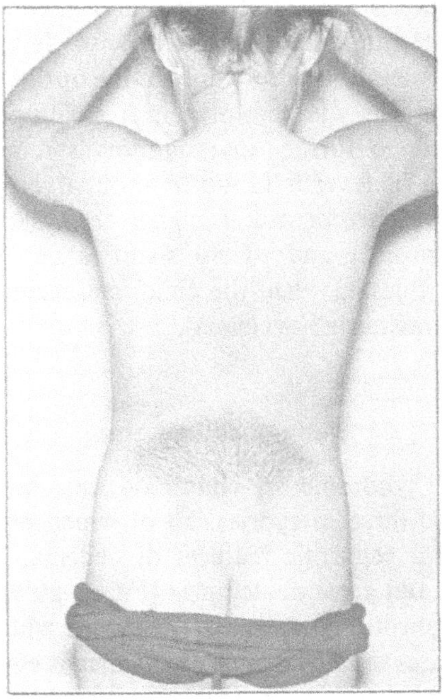

Figure 10.7. *A lumbar hairy patch overlying a closed neural tube defect.*

sore throat, haematuria, oliguria, hypertension, and mild to moderate facial oedema, is even rarer. The child usually presents with only one or two of these and often without clinical, historical or serological evidence of preceding haemolytic streptococcal infection (Meadow 1975). Children with this condition should be admitted to hospital for investigation and treatment. The prognosis for acute post-streptococcal glomerulonephritis is good, but it may take up to two years for the haematuria to clear completely. In non-streptococcal glomerulonephritis, the outcome is more variable and some of these children progress to chronic nephritis.

Chronic Glomerulonephritis

Haematuria is a frequent finding, though rarely the presenting symptom of chronic glomerulonephritis (see West and McAdams 1978). The child may present in the acute phase of nephritis, which fails to resolve, or with the nephrotic syndrome, proteinuria, hypertension or growth failure due to renal failure. Such patients require full investigation as shown in Table 10.5 and will not be considered further.

Focal Glomerulonephritis

Focal glomerulonephritis is one of the commonest causes of renal haematuria. Typically, the child presents

Table 10.4. Causes of haematuria in childhood.

Local causes: e.g. meatal ulcer, perineal excoriation
Urinary tract infection
Congenital malformations (e.g. hydronephrosis)
Focal glomerulonephritis/benign haematuria
Acute nephritis
Chronic glomerulonephritis
Henoch—Schönlein purpura
Calculus
Haemolytic—uraemic syndrome
Polycystic kidneys
Trauma
Renal vein thrombosis
Haemorrhagic diathesis
Septicaemia, subacute bacterial endocarditis
Tumour—benign/malignant
Drugs—especially sulphonamides

Table 10.5. Investigation of haematuria.

Routine investigation
FBC, ESR and platelets
MSU
Throat swab
Blood culture
Urea, electrolytes and creatinine
Calcium, phosphorus, alkaline phosphatase
Plasma proteins and electrophoretic strip
Complement levels
ASO titre
IVU
Subsequent investigation, if indicated
Urinary electrolytes, calcium, urea, uric acid, protein, cystine
Clotting studies
Ultrasound scan
Cystoscopy
Renal biopsy
Micturating cystourethrography

with heavy haematuria but is clinically well. There may have been a triggering respiratory infection and quite commonly there is mild loin or abdominal pain; the attacks are often precipitated by exercise. The routine tests listed in Table 10.5 are normal apart from the haematuria. Many subsequent similar attacks of haematuria may occur. They usually last for a period of 24 to 48 hours (as far as *macroscopic* haematuria is concerned). The attacks may recur every two to three months but they tend to become less common as the child gets older, although in some the disease persists

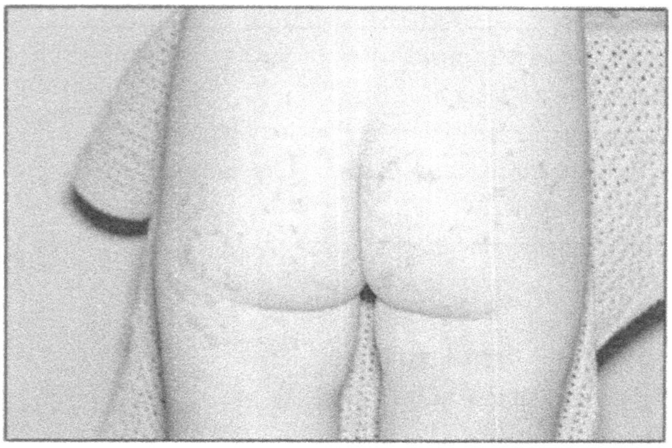

Figure 10.8. *Henoch-Schönlein purpura. A typical petechial and maculopapular rash on the buttocks.*

into adult life. As long as the urine clears completely between episodes of haematuria, and there is no persistent proteinuria, the condition is benign and no further investigation is required. If the haematuria is persistent, or is associated with other clinical or biochemical abnormalities in the presence of a normal IVU, then a renal biopsy should be carried out. In focal glomerulonephritis there is little histological abnormality apart from small areas of increased cellularity in the mesangium of some glomeruli, but in many cases immunofluorescent techniques show widespread IgA deposition in glomerular tufts. The implication of this finding and the aetiology of the condition remain obscure. However, the prognosis is good and the child can usually be spared complex investigations and biopsy.

Proteinuria

Proteinuria has been discussed by West (1976). The main causes in childhood are listed in Table 10.6.

Table 10.6. Causes of proteinuria in childhood.

Orthostatic
Fever—nonspecific
Nephrotic syndrome
Chronic glomerulonephritis or pyelonephritis
UTI (uncommonly causes proteinuria)
Many of the causes of haematuria listed in Table 10.4:
a) because of protein in blood
b) because of underlying pathology
'Adult' disorders—all rare in children, e.g. diabetic nephropathy

Orthostatic and Febrile Causes

The commonest causes of proteinuria in childhood are orthostatic and that associated with fever. In the former, proteinuria occurs only in the upright position, and early morning urine is protein free. The condition is benign and no further investigation is required. The proteinuria of fever is found in about five per cent of children with temperatures higher than 38.5°C. It is usually transient and of no significance. The urine should be retested when the child is afebrile to ensure that the proteinuria has cleared.

Nephrotic Syndrome

Nephrotic syndrome in childhood can be classified simply into three categories, all of which present with the classical nephrotic features of oedema, hypoalbuminaemia and gross proteinuria (Figure 10.9). By definition, nephrotic syndrome is diagnosed when proteinuria is greater than 40 $mg/m^2/hr$, which is equivalent to about 3 to 4 g per day in a 20 kg child. More protein is usually present in the urine in the acute phase of the disease. Since the proteinuria is orthostatic, there is definite merit in bed rest as this will restrict albumin loss and allow the plasma albumin, and hence the plasma colloid osmotic pressure, to return to normal more rapidly and hasten clearing of the oedema.

Congenital Nephrotic Syndrome

This rare condition presents early in infancy. Full assessment is necessary as it can occasionally be caused by congenital infections, including CMV and syphilis, but in the inherited forms the outcome is uniformly fatal.

Minimal Change Nephrotic Syndrome

This is the classical nephrotic syndrome of childhood, which is rarely associated with haematuria or hypertension, and in which there is no evidence of complement consumption. Histologically, the kidney is normal on light microscopy, but the electron microscope reveals fusion of the foot process of the epithelial cells of Bowman's capsule.

Children with this condition are usually under five years of age at presentation, have a highly selective proteinuria (i.e. rarely leak molecules larger than those of albumin into the urine), and almost always go into remission on steroid therapy. Once in remission and free from proteinuria, the child can be allowed home and the steroid dosage gradually reduced over several weeks. An alternate day dosage regime minimizes the toxic side-effects of the steroids.

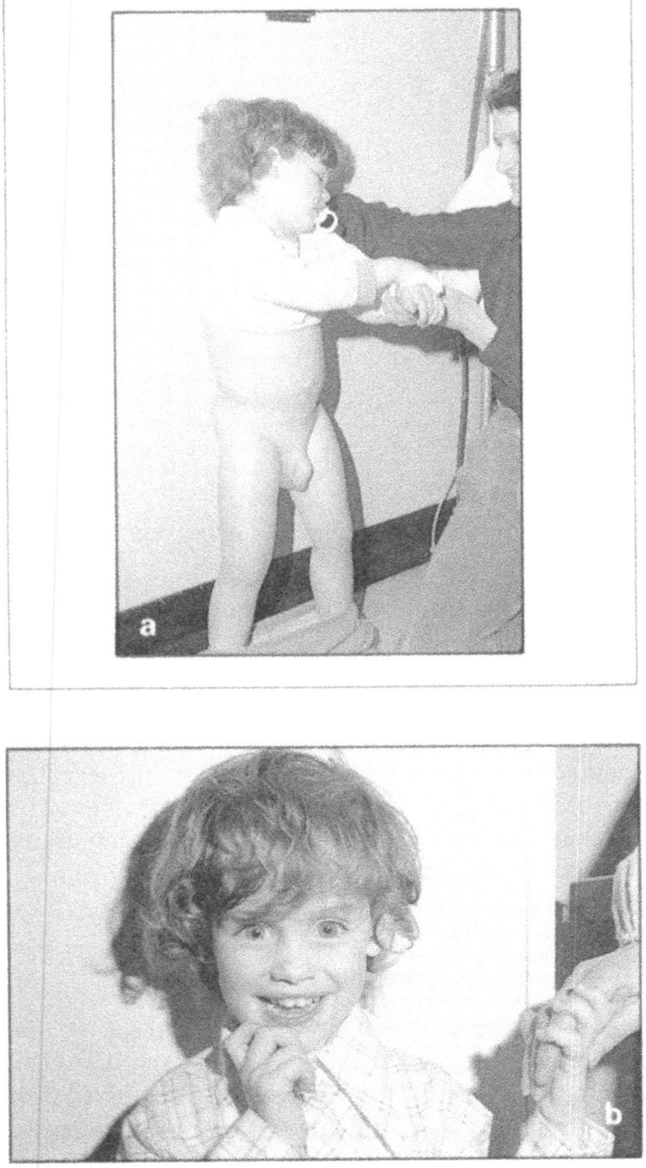

Figure 10.9. *a) A child with nephrotic syndrome showing generalized oedema. b) The same child after recovery.*

Less than 50 per cent of children with minimal change nephrotic syndrome have a sustained remission following steroids; those who relapse usually respond to further courses of steroids, but if relapses persist, or large doses are required to keep the child's urine protein free, cyclophosphamide may be used. This may induce prolonged remission but carries the hazard of gonadal damage, particularly in males, and there is anxiety that this immunosuppressive drug may predispose to malignant disease later in life.

Other Causes of Nephrotic Syndrome

Other causes include all the various types of chronic glomerulonephritis, for which the histopathologists delight in developing ever more complex classifications (West and McAdams 1978). These are of importance in assessing prognosis, and renal biopsy should be carried out, but they are rarely of therapeutic relevance in the acute phase of the illness. Unlike those with minimal change nephrotic syndrome, affected children are typically over five years of age at diagnosis and show associated haematuria and complement consumption. They have non-selective proteinuria and rarely respond to steroids. Remission can often be induced by bed rest, infusions of albumin and diuretics. The aim of therapy is to maintain the patient free from the nephrotic state by maintaining albumin synthesis at a level exceeding loss. The disease process may then 'burn itself out', leaving the child with a variable degree of kidney damage which may be compatible with a reasonably good long-term outlook. If this cannot be achieved the prognosis is very poor.

Persisting Non-orthostatic, Non-nephrotic Proteinuria

Haematuria is, of course, associated with loss into the urine of blood proteins as well as cells. To check whether there is an excess loss of protein, a 'haematocrit' can be carried out on a freshly passed specimen of urine. From this, the amount of protein expected from the blood loss can be calculated. In patients with proteinuria, a wide variety of abnormalities may be present, but if there are no other symptoms, such as those of UTI, and there is no associated haematuria, then the most likely diagnosis is some form of chronic nephritis. In addition to assessment of the degree and selectivity of the proteinuria, the tests for haematuria listed in Table 10.5 should be performed.

Conclusion

It is apparent that in childhood renal tract disease the application of good diagnostic methods and prompt, appropriate treatment will not only relieve a great deal of unnecessary suffering, but will help also to reduce the number of children—two to three per million total population per year—who develop chronic renal failure.

References

Meadow, S. R., *Arch. Dis. Childh.*, 1975, **50**, 379.

Smellie, J. M. and Normand, I. C. S., Urinary tract infection with and without anatomic malformations, in: *Clinical Paediatric Nephrology*, Ed. E. J. B. Liebermann, Lippincott, 1976, p.194.

West, C. J., *J. Pediatr.*, 1976, **89**, 173.

West, C. D. and McAdams, A. J., *J. Pediatr.*, 1978, **93**, 1 and 167.

Further Reading

James, J. A., *Renal Disease in Childhood*, Mosby, St. Louis, 1976.

Liebermann, E. J. B. (Ed.), *Clinical Paediatric Nephrology*, Lippincott, 1976.

11. Gut Problems

GASTROINTESTINAL symptoms account for a considerable proportion of childhood general practice consultations. Fortunately, most of this disease is mild and self-limiting and is best managed by reassurance and masterly inactivity. The prudent doctor, however, always bears in mind how very quickly an apparently well child can become desperately ill. This is especially true of infants who are losing fluid and it is essential to keep them under close observation.

In this chapter we will discuss common gut problems, largely in terms of their presenting symptoms.

Gastroenteritis

Gastroenteritis (see McClung 1978) remains a major cause of infant morbidity and mortality even in highly developed countries. In England and Wales it accounts for approximately 10 per cent of all medical paediatric admissions and between 200 and 300 deaths annually. It is most serious in children under the age of two years, in whom dehydration may develop very rapidly. Indeed, profound dehydration from fluid loss into the gut lumen may occasionally occur before vomiting or diarrhoea is evident. It is therefore of the greatest importance that the clinical symptoms and signs of fluid loss are recognized. These are:

1. Weight loss. A recent weight recording is often available for infants who attend a Welfare Clinic regularly, and this may permit an accurate, objective assessment of fluid loss to be made.
2. Decreased urinary output. This is often apparent to the mothers of babies in nappies.
3. Thirst.
4. Dry mouth.
5. Decreased skin turgor. This generally reliable sign may be misleading in hypernatraemic dehydration, in which the skin has an odd doughy consistency, and in fat infants.
6. Sunken anterior fontanelle, sunken eyes and decreased eyeball turgor.
7. Tachypnoea due to metabolic acidosis.
8. Tachycardia.
9. Shock.

Loss of skin turgor becomes detectable when the child is about 2.5 to 5 per cent dehydrated, i.e. has lost that proportion of his body weight in water. Obvious signs are apparent at 10 per cent dehydration, and frank shock at around 15 per cent.

Differential Diagnosis

Many childhood infections, especially those of the respiratory tract, present with vomiting and diarrhoea due to the general systemic upset, often combined with the effects of swallowing infected mucus. Conversely, gastroenteritis may be mistaken for serious respiratory disease because of the acidosis-induced hyperventilation. Careful examination will usually avoid these errors in diagnosis.

Aetiology

Gastroenteritis is caused by bacteria, including enteropathogenic *E. coli*, *Salmonella*, *Shigella* and the more recently recognized *Campylobacter*, and by viruses, particularly the Rotavirus (Figure 11.1). The clinical syndrome tends to show characteristic features for each of these pathogens, as summarized in Table 11.1.

Treatment

Children with mild gastroenteritis can be managed at home, but those with more than 5 per cent dehydration require hospital admission.

Table 11.1. Typical clinical features of the common causes of gastroenteritis.

	Shigella	*E. coli*	*Salmonella*	*Campylobacter*	Rotavirus
Age	6 mths–5 years	Under 2 years	Any	Any	Under 2 years
Seasons	◄————	Usually late summer	————	————►	Winter
Diarrhoea in household	50%	No	Variable	Variable (including pets)	Variable
Incubation	24–72 hours	24–48 hours	8–24 hours	2–5 days	48–72 hours
Vomiting	Absent	±	Common	±	Common
High fever	Common	Absent	±	±	Common
Respiratory symptoms	25%	Absent	Absent	Absent	URTI common
Fits	10%	Rare	Rare	Absent	Absent
Pain	Common	Rare	Variable	Marked	Rare
Stools					
Consistency	Watery	Loose	Loose slimy	Watery	Watery
Blood	±	–	–	+	–
Mucus	+	±	±	±	–
Pus	+	–	–	–	–

Rehydration Procedure

The aim of treatment at home should be to give clear fluids by mouth in sufficient volume and with sufficient frequency to correct dehydration, and then to sustain hydration without inducing further vomiting. Precise instructions must always be given about the amount and type of fluid recommended. Misunderstood casual instructions about pinches of salt, spoonfuls of sugar and unspecified quantities of fluid can result in emetic mixtures of bizarre chemical composition which are, at best, ineffective and, at worst, dangerous. We have seen irreversible hypernatraemia in a child with mild gastroenteritis whose mother was directed, by a doctor's receptionist, to give her boiled water with one teaspoonful of sugar and one teaspoonful of salt to the pint.

Figure 11.1. *Rotavirus, now recognized as a common cause of gastroenteritis in children.*

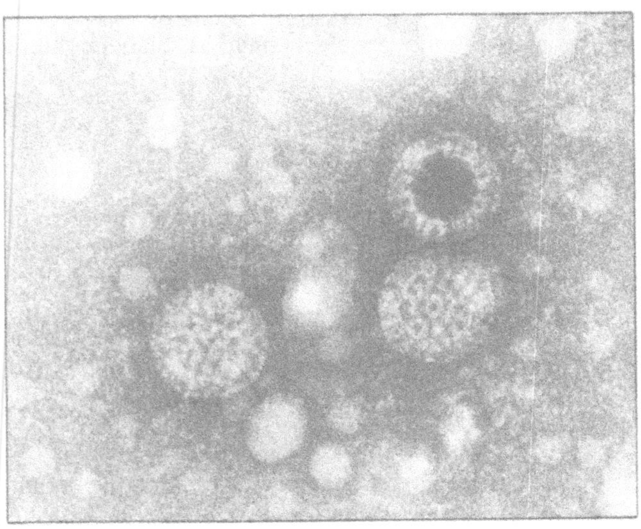

Suitable rehydration fluids. Rehydration fluid of suitable composition for infants and children can best be prepared using either Dioralyte sachets, one to 200 ml of water, or Electrosol tablets, also one to 200 ml of water. Dioralyte contains sugar (as dextrose) but Electrosol does not. The composition of these preparations is given in Table 11.2. A less satisfactory, but safe and usually acceptable, alternative is provided by the ubiquitous Coca Cola diluted to quarter or half strength. Failing these, lightly flavoured and sweetened water without salt is recommended. At least 150 to 200 ml of fluid per kg per 24 hours should be given, divided into small amounts and administered at frequent intervals to minimize vomiting.

Managed in this way vomiting and diarrhoea will usually stop within 24 hours. Gradual regrading of infants' feeds can then be undertaken along the lines suggested in Table 11.3. Older infants with less severe gastroenteritis can often be regraded more rapidly and, in those over two years of age, light foods such as jelly, ice cream or dry toast can be used to reintroduce solids within 24 hours.

Treatment of Recurrent Symptoms

Recurrence of symptoms during the regrading process is best managed by a brief return to clear fluids. In about five per cent of children with severe gastroenteritis, recovery is delayed by recurrent diarrhoea when milk is restarted. This is frequently due to lactose intolerance resulting from damage to the delicate lactase-containing

Table 11.2. Composition of electrolyte solutions.

	Dioralyte (5 sachets/litre water) (mmol/l)	Electrosol BP (5 tabs/litre water) (mmol/l)
Sodium	35	29
Potassium	20	10.5
Chloride	37	28
Bicarbonate	18	12
Dextrose	200 (mg/dl)	nil

epithelial cells of the small intestine. The stool is characteristically acid due to the presence of organic acids derived from lactose, and the presence of a reducing sugar—unaltered lactose—can be demonstrated in the stool supernatant with Clinitest tablets. In such infants, the diarrhoea responds to removal of lactose from the diet by using a lactose-free milk preparation such as Velactin, Nutramigen or Galactomin. Occasionally, persistent diarrhoea may be due to cows' milk protein intolerance; such infants require a milk based on soya bean protein, such as Velactin. Fortunately, secondary lactose and protein intolerance are usually transient and normal feeding can be reintroduced after a few weeks.

Use of Antibiotics

Antibiotics should not be used in uncomplicated gastroenteritis due to *Salmonella, Shigella* or *E. coli,* since they tend to prolong the carrier state, or in viral gastroenteritis because they merely encourage gut superinfection with other organisms. *Campylobacter* infections should probably be treated with oral erythromycin. If there is clinical suspicion of septicaemia in association with gastroenteritis, the child should be admitted to hospital and treated with appropriate antibiotics intravenously.

Table 11.3. Scheme for regrading of feeds following gastroenteritis.

		Regrading by quarters (ml/kg corrected weight/day)	Regrading by fifths (ml/kg corrected weight/day)
Day 1	GEM[1]	150	150
Day 2	GEM	115	120
	Milk feeding	35	30
Day 3	GEM	75	90
	Milk feeding	75	60
Day 4	GEM	35	60
	Milk feeding	115	90
Day 5	GEM	—	30
	Milk feeding	150	120

[1] GEM = glucose-electrolyte mixture.
From Walker Smith 1975 with permission.

Use of Antiemetics and Antidiarrhoeals

Antiemetic and antidiarrhoeal agents have no place in the management of infantile gastroenteritis. They are ineffective and produce a high incidence of side-effects. In older children, they may provide useful symptomatic relief but should also be used sparingly. We are particularly wary of the phenothiazines and allied drugs (e.g. Stemetil, Fentazin and Maxolon), because of the unpleasant dystonic reactions they may cause.

Vomiting

Innumerable conditions in childhood may present with vomiting as the primary symptom. Some of the more important of these will be considered, and subdivided along the lines of our own diagnostic thought processes.

Acute Vomiting

With Fever

In addition to gastroenteritis, almost any infection may present with acute vomiting and fever. In young children, the more important to bear in mind include respiratory tract infections, especially otitis media, urinary tract infection, appendicitis and meningitis.

Without Fever

Acute vomiting without fever may be due to food poisoning, ingestion of drugs or toxins, psychological and behavioural problems, migraine, the periodic syndrome, intestinal obstruction, raised intracranial pressure or a metabolic problem such as diabetic ketoacidosis.

Persistent Vomiting

Persistent vomiting is an extremely common problem in paediatrics. In its evaluation it is important to know, or to ascertain as soon as possible, whether the child is growing and gaining weight at a satisfactory rate.

Persistent Vomiting with Normal Growth and Weight Gain

This problem is most frequently due to simple reflux vomiting or regurgitation, which presumably reflects relative incompetence of the infantile cardiac sphincter. Typically, the baby regurgitates small amounts of milk throughout the day and especially after feeds when winded. He is free from other symptoms and entirely unperturbed, although the trail of small but smelly vomits he leaves in his path may provoke his house-proud mother to consider infanticide! No investigation is required because, even if a small hiatus hernia is demonstrated, no special measures are needed in a thriving child without evidence of peptic oesophagitis. The problem resolves with remarkable constancy around the end of the first year, when the child starts to get up on his feet. Until this time symptomatic relief can be achieved by avoiding overfilling the baby's stomach, winding him carefully, keeping him propped up for some time after feeds and by thickening the feeds with an unabsorbed preparation, such as Nestargel or Carobel (one scoop per 120 ml of milk). The parents must be reassured and told of the natural history of the condition.

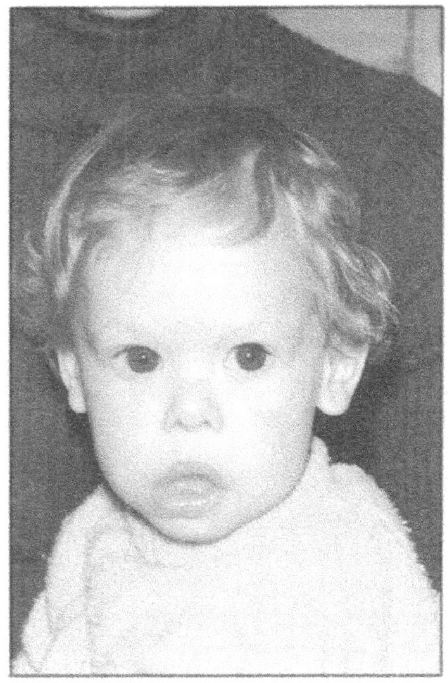

Figure 11.2. *A boy, aged 18 months, who presented with persistent vomiting, failure to thrive and retarded development. His 'elfin' face is typical of infantile hypercalcaemia, which was confirmed chemically.*

Persistent Vomiting with Inadequate Growth or Weight Gain

The more important conditions to consider are listed in Table 11.4 (see Figure 11.2). Hospital admission is generally required for full assessment of these problems.

Diarrhoea

It is important to ascertain whether the problem is excessive frequency or excessive looseness of the stools. Once again the significance of the symptom is generally assessed according to the growth and weight gain of the child. Although normal growth strongly suggests that serious underlying disease is not present, children may occasionally continue to grow and gain weight adequately despite gastrointestinal disease, probably because of a compensatory increase in caloric intake. Persistent diarrhoea due to chronic bacterial infection of the gut is rare in the UK, and, therefore, stool culture seldom proves helpful in diagnosis. The major causes of persistent diarrhoea are listed in Table 11.5 (see Figures 11.3 and 11.4). Spurious diarrhoea complicating constipation is particularly common and can be detected easily by rectal examination.

When all the conditions in Table 11.5 have been excluded, a large number of children, who pass up to four loose stools daily but continue to grow normally, remain bereft of a diagnosis. By the age of four years, the stool pattern has generally become more normal. An interesting recent hypothesis ascribes the problem to inadequate fat intake (Cohen et al. 1978).

Table 11.4. Causes of persistent vomiting with weight loss.

Congenital hypertrophic pyloric stenosis
Hiatus hernia, achalasia cardia
Rumination
Chronic infection, e.g. tuberculosis, urinary tract infection, hepatitis
Whooping cough
Coeliac disease
Cows' milk protein intolerance
Raised intracranial pressure, e.g. subdural haematoma, benign intracranial hypertension
Metabolic problems, e.g. diabetes, galactosaemia, congenital adrenal hyperplasia, hypercalcaemia
Uraemia

Rectal Bleeding

Fresh Blood in the Stool

Anal fissure is common and is the usual cause of fresh blood on the stool associated with painful defaecation. The fissure is usually visible at the posterior anal margin. The stools must be softened to allow healing and local anaesthetic jelly can be used for defaecation.

Fresh blood and mucus, said typically to resemble red-currant jelly, in the stool of a child with colicky

Table 11.5. Causes of persistent diarrhoea.

Nonspecific diarrhoea
Irritable colon
Spurious diarrhoea with constipation
Carbohydrate intolerance
Emotional stress
Infestation, e.g. giardiasis
Coeliac disease
Fibrocystic disease
Milk protein or other food allergy
Drugs
Rare causes—these are very numerous and include gut malformations, Hirschsprung's disease, Crohn's disease, ulcerative colitis, thyrotoxicosis, functioning neural tumours, etc.

abdominal pain always raises the possibility of intussusception, and immediate hospital admission is necessary for diagnosis and treatment (see chapter 12).

Rectal bleeding in association with diarrhoeal illness suggests *Shigella* or *Campylobacter* enteritis, amoebic dysentery or, possibly, ulcerative colitis.

Painless rectal bleeding may indicate Meckel's diverticulum, a lower intestinal polyp or occasionally a bleeding diathesis. The child should be referred to hospital for investigation.

Figure 11.3. *A boy, aged six years, who presented with chronic diarrhoea, abdominal distension and growth failure. He was found to have coeliac disease.*

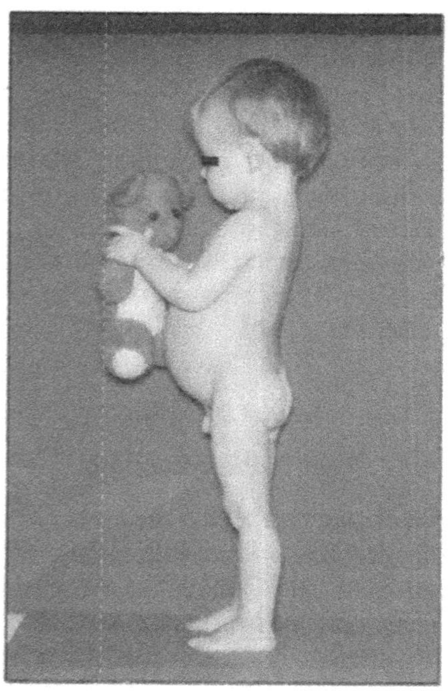

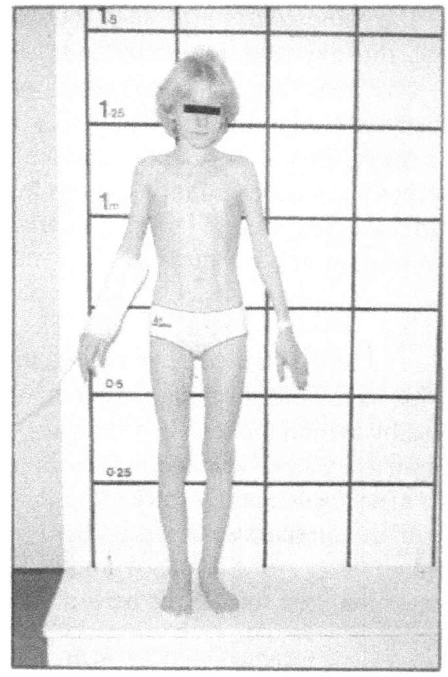

Figure 11.4. *A girl, aged 12 years, who presented with chronic diarrhoea, recurrent chest infections and growth failure. She was found to have fibrocystic disease.*

Melaena

Melaena is an unusual symptom in an otherwise well child. Most cases occur in the presence of known disease, such as portal hypertension or peptic ulceration. The bleeding from a Meckel's diverticulum may also present as melaena and simpler explanations, such as drug-induced gastritis and swallowed blood, must not be forgotten.

Constipation

Are the stools too hard, too infrequent, or both? There is great variation in normal bowel habit, especially in breast-fed babies who may pass several stools daily or one weekly.

Constipation in childhood is very rarely due to serious organic disease, such as Hirschsprung's disease or an unrecognized spinal lesion, and when these are present clinical clues, such as the neonatal onset of problems, the intractable nature of the constipation or the presence of other neurological abnormalities, will usually alert the vigilant doctor.

Chronic Constipation

Chronic constipation in childhood is nearly always the end result of a familiar vicious circle of events. During a febrile illness the child becomes slightly dehydrated and the stools are hard. The passage of a large hard stool causes an anal fissure so defaecation becomes acutely painful. The child is then very reasonably disinclined to open his bowels and withholds as long as he possibly can. The large hard stool he eventually passes aggravates his fissure and further convinces him that this highly undesirable activity must be postponed as long as possible! Frequently, not only the rectum but most of the colon becomes enormously dilated with hard faeces, and spurious diarrhoea and soiling results from leakage around the faecal masses. Psychological disturbance is much more frequently a secondary result of the social distress and embarrassment so caused than it is the primary event causing the constipation.

To break the vicious circle it is first necessary to empty the colon and rectum. One or two enemas are occasionally needed but Dulcolax suppositories are almost as effective and more acceptable. Once this initial emptying has been achieved, a good diet including plenty of fluid and unabsorbed roughage must be established and regular laxatives given. The combination of a colonic stimulant and a stool softener is effective. We favour Senokot, as tablets, granules or syrup, and Dioctyl-Medo (dioctyl sodium sulphosuccinate) syrup. The parents can be instructed to adjust the dose of each to give a regular, soft stool. With long-established constipation, treatment must be given for several months, after which it is nearly always possible to wean the child gradually from the medication. Simple behaviour modification techniques, such as a star chart with suitable rewards, often help the retraining process. Soiling in association with constipation nearly always responds to this regime and we seldom find it necessary to proceed to anal dilatation with a general anaesthetic (Clayden and Lawson 1976).

Deliberate soiling in a child with a normal bowel habit is a different matter and frequently indicates serious psychological disturbance which merits full psychiatric evaluation.

Worms

Threadworms

Infestation with the threadworm, or pinworm, *Enteriobius vermicularis* is very common in the UK. The ova are shed onto the perianal skin by the female worm and are then spread by the anus-finger-mouth route of transmission.

The usual presentation is nocturnal perianal pruritus, but it is important to remember that the worms can migrate to the introitus of little girls and cause vulvovaginitis, which may in turn cause dysuria.

The diagnosis is confirmed either by spotting worms at the anal margin early in the morning or by the Sellotape swab technique, in which a piece of Sellotape is applied to the anal margin first thing in the morning and is then stuck down onto a microscope slide. Threadworm ova can then be identified.

Although piperazine compounds have been the traditional treatment for this infestation they are not invariably successful, and when given in too large a dose are a potent cause of ataxia—the 'worm wobble'. Mebendazole (Vermox) has become the drug of choice; one 100 mg tablet should be given not only to the patient but to all members of the family. In addition, it is essential to launder thoroughly all bedclothes, underwear and night clothes and to give instructions about personal hygiene, in particular cleaning under the fingernails. A second dose may be given in two or three weeks if necessary.

Ascariasis, Trichuriasis and Ankylostomiasis

These conditions are extremely rare in natives of the UK, but are seen increasingly among immigrant children. Ascariasis and trichuriasis are usually asymptomatic, and are only detected clinically when worms are passed per rectum or, in the case of ascariasis, appear through the mouth or nostrils. Ova can be seen in the stool on microscopy. Ankylostomiasis may cause abdominal pain and an iron deficiency anaemia. It is also diagnosed by demonstrating the typical ova in the stools. All three conditions can be treated with mebendazole 100 mg b.d. for three days.

Tape Worms

With today's high standards of meat preparation, tapeworm infestation is rare. It is usually asymptomatic but proglottids may be passed in the faeces. The condition can be treated with niclosamide (Yomesan).

References

Clayden, G. S. and Lawson, J. O. N., *Arch. Dis. Childh.*, 1976, **51**, 918.

Cohen, S., Lake, A. M., Mathis, R. K. and Walker, W. A., *Pediatrics*, 1978, **61**, 808.

McClung, H. J., *Etiology, Pathophysiology and Treatment of Acute Gastroenteritis*, Report of the 74th Ross conference on pediatric research, Ross Laboratories, Columbus, Ohio, USA, 1978.

Further Reading

Anderson, C. M. and Burke, V., *Paediatric Gastroenterology*, Blackwell, Oxford, 1975.

Walker Smith, J., *Diseases of the Small Intestine in Childhood*, Pitman Medical, Tunbridge Wells, 1975, p. 143.

12. Abdominal Pain

ABDOMINAL pain is arguably the most difficult of all the common childhood symptoms to evaluate. Experience and care in the approach to this problem fail to bring immunity from rude surprises! Joseph Brenneman, one of the most famous of American paediatricians, wrote: 'After 40 years' extensive experience I still approach the painful abdomen of a child with much apprehension and a greater feeling of uncertainty than any other domain of childhood'. It is an area in which it is essential to be cautious and to leave a wide margin for diagnostic error but as long as we remain acutely aware that this is a minefield through which it is our aim to take the most prudent rather than the shortest route, we should be able to manage children presenting in this way safely and, usually, successfully.

Much of the writing on abdominal pain in childhood seems to us to suffer from the attempt to be comprehensive. Although the possible causes are legion, those that appear regularly in the wards we share with our paediatric surgical colleagues comprise no more than an undermanned cohort! We are still searching, for instance, with somewhat tarnished enthusiasm, for a case of acute intermittent porphyria presenting in this way, and we seldom see conditions common in other parts of the world, such as lead poisoning and sickle cell disease. Therefore, we will confine our attention to problems relatively commonly seen in England. Failure to recognize common conditions presenting in an unusual way is a far more frequent source of diagnostic error than is failure to consider rare conditions.

The problem of the child seen as an emergency with acute abdominal pain is obviously different from that presented by the 'little bellyacher' with recurrent bouts of pain, so we will consider these two major categories separately.

Acute Abdominal Pain

We have already established that, faced with a child with acute abdominal pain, our objective is to make not a full diagnosis but a sensible clinical decision. The problem is different for each of the three doctors involved: the general practitioner must decide whether the child should stay at home or be admitted to hospital; the surgeon must decide whether to perform a laparotomy; and the paediatrician must decide whether the pain is due to a treatable disease. Often the general practitioner, who is the first in line, can answer all three questions, and he can almost always supply information which is extremely helpful to the others.

The first essential is, of course, as full and careful a history and physical examination as the circumstances allow. One point seems worthy of special emphasis: as generations of MB examiners have been at pains to impress on us, testing the urine is an essential part of the examination. Spare a thought for your forebears inadvertently splashing themselves with smelly boiling urine from burping test tubes and dip your simple, hygienic and extremely informative Multistix into this most painlessly acquired of vital fluids! If you cannot obtain any urine before sending a child to hospital we would advise noting the fact in your letter to remind your fallible hospital colleagues, tactfully, that many a child with diabetic ketoacidosis, hepatitis or pyelonephritis has had his urine tested after his laparotomy!

In Figure 12.1 we have outlined an approach to the child with acute abdominal pain. Let us consider the choices offered.

Extra- or Intra-abdominal?

First, is the pain truly within the abdomen or is it referred from an extra-abdominal site? A reasonably confident answer to this question requires specific consideration of the possibility of referred pain during the obligatory general physical examination. Several sites may be involved. Many young children complain of abdominal pain when the only objective finding is an upper respiratory tract infection. Some, but probably not all, have significant intra-abdominal gland enlarge-

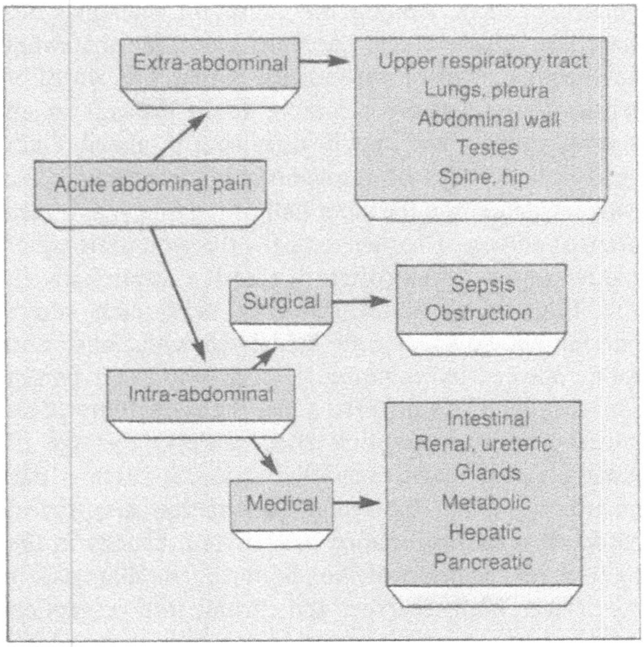

Figure 12.1. *Causes of acute abdominal pain in childhood.*

ment and so belong to the mesenteric adenitis group. Disease of the lower respiratory tract is particularly liable to cause confusion when the diaphragmatic pleura, especially on the right side, is inflamed by basal pneumonia. The abdominal wall is a frequent source of pain, and sometimes tenderness, after local trauma, violent vomiting or coughing, and in association with viral infections, especially pleurodynia. The testes must never be forgotten, torsion particularly is a danger at any age and pain from this site is frequently referred to the central or lower abdomen. Finally, pain originating in the spine or hip may cause confusion.

Surgical Problems

Second, having decided that the pain is intra-abdominal in origin, is it surgical or medical? Surgical problems requiring immediate operation are essentially those of sepsis and obstruction. The possibility of pelvic disease must be considered, particularly in the adolescent girl, but other surgical conditions are rare.

Intra-abdominal Sepsis

Severity, persistence and localization of the pain are all ominous features but the cardinal sign of intra-abdominal sepsis is tenderness in association with fever. Although sometimes necessary, it is extremely difficult to feel the abdomen of a child who is sitting on his mother's lap or, indeed, in any position other than lying supine and reasonably relaxed. Most children can be persuaded to lie down and, unless the pain is both severe and continuous, to take an interest in something else while the examiner explores gently for tenderness, watching the child's face for clues to the site and degree of pain elicited. A simple test for the presence of sepsis which sometimes proves useful is the 'jump test'. The principle of this is that an enthusiastic standing jump is incompatible with a septic focus in the abdomen. It is remarkable, and most reassuring, how many children who seem to be in quite severe pain, are willing to attempt the All England standing high jump record! Indeed, sometimes the mere fact of being asked to do something so delightful has a powerful therapeutic effect on a child who, minutes before, was prostrate. Caution, as always, must be exercised in interpreting this physical sign; one of the authors recalls with embarrassment an eight-year-old haemophiliac boy who performed a creditable elevation six hours before his acutely inflamed appendix was removed!

A further clue to the presence of sepsis is a neutrophil leucocytosis, especially if the cells show a left shift and toxic granulation.

Appendicitis is by far the most common and most important cause of intra-abdominal sepsis in children. Although it is rare under the age of three years, it always enters the differential diagnosis. Unfortunately, the classical history and findings are the exception rather than the rule, especially in the younger age-group. It is remarkable how often initially obscure symptoms prove to be due to appendicitis. Delay in diagnosis is associated with a greatly increased incidence of morbidity and indeed mortality, so it is vital to retain a high index of suspicion. In a most useful paper Jackson (1963) reviewed a series of 313 children with appendicitis seen in Newcastle, and analysed when and why diagnostic delay occurred. More than 24 hours passed before the general practitioner was called in 48 per cent of cases and more than 48 hours in 19 per cent. Of the latter group, 83 per cent had perforated their appendices before operation, compared with only 24 per cent of those whose general practitioner was called within 12 hours. Further significant delay sometimes occurred after the children were seen. In 29 per cent the diagnosis was not clear at the general practitioner's first visit and further calls were necessary. Of the children who reached hospital within four hours of the first visit, 38 per cent had perforated their appendices whereas only one of the 36 children whose admission was delayed more than 48 hours after the first visit still retained an unruptured appendix. It was abundantly confirmed that the younger the child the more difficult the diagnosis, but many other factors contributed to diagnostic difficulty. The appendix was in the classical subcaecal site in only 32 per cent of the children, in 27 per cent it was retrocaecal, in 23 per cent pelvic and in 11 per cent at another site. Abdominal tenderness was often slight and sometimes completely absent in children with retrocaecal appendices, and urinary symptoms were prominent in those with pelvic appendices. In only one third of cases was there the classical history of constant pain at first central then settling in the right iliac fossa. In some children the pain was intermittent throughout the illness. Fever, vomiting and bowel disturbance occurred in various patterns. A history of previous attacks of similar pain was present in more than one in 10 of the children and other problems, including respiratory or urinary tract infection and gastroenteritis, were sometimes present coincidentally with the appendicitis. Clearly the only possible rule for childhood appendicitis is that no rules apply!

Intestinal Obstruction

The major clinical features of intestinal obstruction are vomiting, absolute constipation, colic, distension and high-pitched bowel sounds, but their relative prominence varies according to the severity, site and duration of the obstruction. The most useful ancillary investigation is the erect abdominal radiograph which usually shows fluid levels (Figure 12.2) and often indicates the site of the lesion. At all ages a diligent search for a strangulated hernia must be made. A previous laparotomy will, of course, suggest the possibility of adhesions but often an exact diagnosis must await the surgical findings and the clinical problem is simply to suspect obstruction and then to amass enough evidence to leave no doubt that laparotomy is necessary.

Figure 12.2. *The erect abdominal radiograph of an infant who presented with intestinal obstruction after an episode of neonatal necrotizing enterocolitis. Multiple air-fluid levels are shown. At laparotomy a stricture of the descending colon was found.*

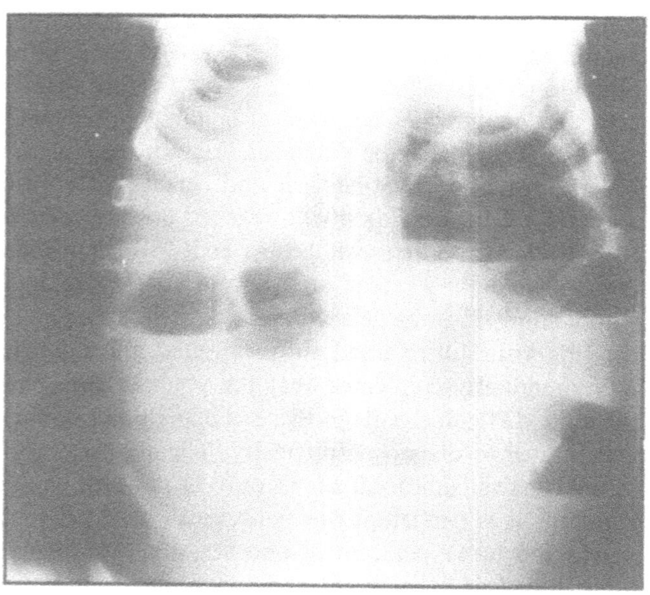

Intussusception. Among the causes of intestinal obstruction, intussusception occupies a position somewhat analogous to that of appendicitis among the causes of sepsis. It is relatively common, often presents in an atypical manner and may be disastrous if missed. Once again a high index of suspicion is vital. Although the peak incidence is in the latter half of the first year it may occur at any age. Characteristically the symptoms are of sudden onset, a well (often, it seems, exceptionally fit and flourishing) infant suddenly developing severe intermittent bouts of colic associated with pallor and soon followed by vomiting. If such symptoms persist for more than two or three hours the probability of an underlying intussusception rises sharply. Passage of blood-stained 'redcurrant jelly' stools is often a late manifestation but the rectal examination may reveal blood. If a sausage-shaped mass is felt, usually in the right upper quadrant of the abdomen, the diagnosis is confirmed. Both recurrent and chronic intussusception may occur, so this diagnosis must not only be entertained in acute illness. Children in whom intussusception is suspected must be observed in hospital. The plain radiograph appearances are often suggestive but the definitive diagnosis requires a barium enema (Figure 12.3) and, especially when the diagnosis has been made early, reduction of the intussusception can often be achieved by hydrostatic pressure at the same examination. This procedure requires an experienced radiologist and, if it fails, laparotomy must be undertaken without delay.

Medical Problems

The renal tract is probably the most frequent site of 'medical' pain of sufficient severity to cause confusion in this context. Acute pyelonephritis often produces severe pain and tenderness, easily mistaken, on the right side, for appendicitis. Examination of the urine should establish the diagnosis but it is important to remember that an inflamed appendix in juxtaposition with the renal tract can elicit both symptoms and microscopic findings suggesting urinary tract infection. Renal colic, from stones or clots, is uncommon.

Pain from the gastrointestinal tract may also be acute and severe, especially in acute gastroenteritis. Henoch-Schönlein disease is surprisingly common and often causes severe abdominal pain. Fortunately, it is unusual for the pain to present before the characteristic purpuric rash (Figure 12.4) or the joint swelling. The possibility of an underlying intussusception must be kept in mind. Other gastrointestinal problems which may present acutely include Crohn's disease and peptic ulceration.

Mesenteric adenitis mimics appendicitis frequently and, indeed, often cannot safely be differentiated from it. A high fever, the presence of upper respiratory tract

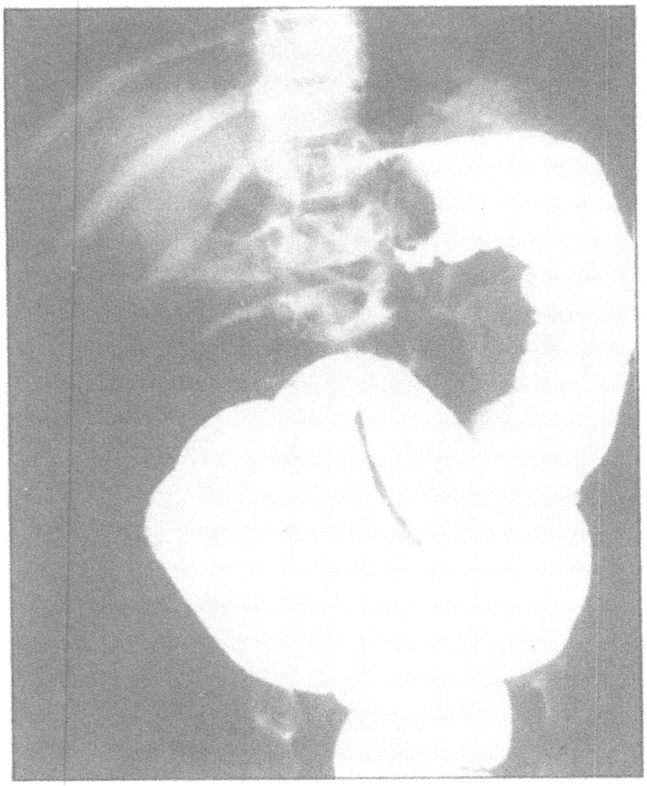

Figure 12.3. *Ileocolic intussusception demonstrated by barium enema in a one-year-old child who presented with a 36-hour history of severe colicky abdominal pain and 'redcurrent jelly' stools. A laparotomy was necessary, but when this important diagnosis is made earlier, reduction can often be achieved by barium enema.*

infection, spasmodic pain and a shifting point of maximal abdominal tenderness are characteristic, but certainly not pathognomic, signs. Other infections, including influenza, infectious mononucleosis and rheumatic fever may cause acute abdominal pain.

Among the metabolic problems which may cause acute pain diabetic ketoacidosis is the most common and most important and must always be excluded.

Hepatitis may present with pain and tenderness in the right upper abdomen. Jaundice is usually, but not always, detectable clinically and the chief clue will then be the presence of urobilinogen and bilirubin in the urine. Pancreatitis is most commonly a feature of mumps, but may occur in other infections and as a side-effect of steroids and other drugs.

Recurrent Abdominal Pain

It is unnecessary to remind general practitioners that this is one of the more persistent and intractable problems in paediatric medicine. Do your spirits sink a little when, at the end of a long surgery, one or more anxious parents tow in a reluctant child and demand that something is done about his endless complaints of tummyache? No doubt the universal acceptance of John Apley's term 'little bellyachers' owed as much to its mildly pejorative as to its purely descriptive qualities!

We are of course indebted to Apley for much more than this useful term, because his monograph *The Child with Abdominal Pains,* first published in 1959, remains the classic account of the epidemiology, clinical aspects and management of the problem and, indeed, much of what follows is derived from it. For the purposes of his studies he included children who were more than three years old and, during a period of more than three months, had more than three attacks of pain of sufficient severity to disturb their activity. The incidence of such symptoms in children of school age was approximately 10 per cent overall, a little higher in girls and lower in boys. Some subsequent surveys have suggested an even higher incidence up to 15 per cent. After careful and thorough investigation of a series of children presenting with this complaint at a hospital outpatient clinic, Apley was able to demonstrate organic disease in only one child in 20. Nevertheless, careful exclusion of organic disease is essential in every case, not only to avoid missing treatable disease in the minority but also because, as discussed below, this is an important and reassuring step in the approach to the majority in whom an organic cause is not demonstrable.

In Table 12.1 we have listed the organic problems which seem to us to occur in this context with sufficient

Figure 12.4. *Henoch-Schönlein purpura. A typical petechial and maculopapular rash on the lower limbs.*

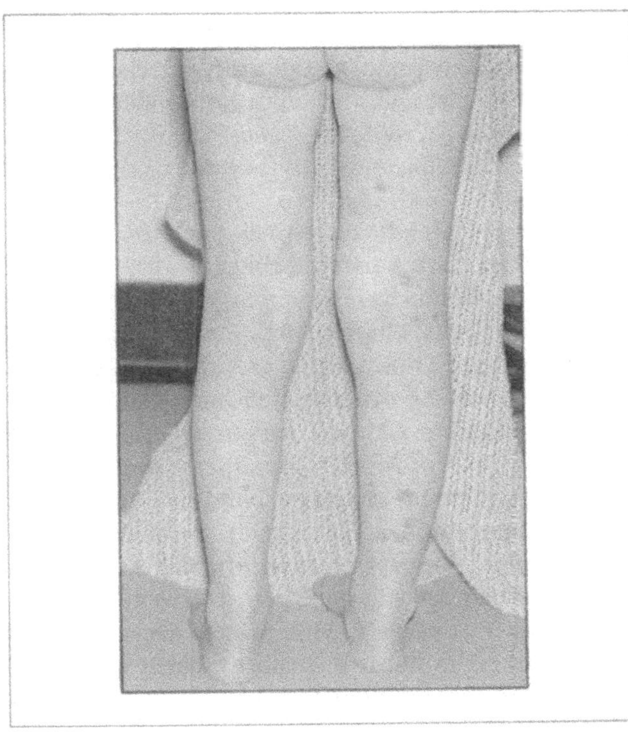

Table 12.1. Organic causes of recurrent abdominal pain.

Renal tract	Recurrent infection
	Hydronephrosis
	Vesicoureteric reflux
	Stone or clot colic
Gastrointestinal tract	Peptic ulcer
	Crohn's disease
	Milk or other food intolerance
	Cholecystitis
Genital tract	Dysmenorrhoea
	Ovulation pain
Intra-abdominal glands	Mesenteric adenitis

frequency to justify inclusion among the relatively commonplace rather than the exotic. In most reported series, renal tract problems have made up the largest group. Clinical clues would, of course, include any history of disturbance of micturition and any abnormality of the urine. Sometimes neither may be present. The 12-year-old boy whose radiographs are shown in Figure 12.5 presented with a history of bouts of abdominal pain for several years but denied any associated symptoms. His parents were anxious and he seemed somewhat hypochondriacal. There were no abnormal physical findings and the urine was normal in all respects. The excellent paediatrician who saw him (neither of the authors) was, however, alerted by the fact that he localized his pain to the right side of the abdomen, and she therefore arranged an IVU (Figure 12.5a). The conclusion to this story is related in the caption. This case admirably illustrates a clinical axiom which has been called Apley's rule, 'The further the site of the pain from the umbilicus the more likely it is to be organic'.

Disease of the gastrointestinal tract usually offers clinical clues to the careful clinician. Children with peptic ulcers seldom have symptoms as clearly related to eating as do adults, but there are often affected relatives in the family. The boy whose radiograph is shown in Figure 12.6 was the son and grandson of ulcer victims (Zollinger-Ellison syndrome was strongly suspected but excluded). Children with Crohn's disease often have not only gastrointestinal symptoms but also a considerable degree of constitutional illness and growth failure.

The role of dietary intolerance in the aetiology of abdominal pain remains uncertain. Milk is the foodstuff most frequently suspect. Milk protein allergy is a well established entity but is difficult to diagnose with certainty except in severely affected children and it seems unlikely to be a frequent cause of obscure abdominal pain. It has recently been suggested, however, that lactose intolerance, due to the normal maturational decline in intestinal lactase activity, may be a very common cause of recurrent pain (Barr et al. 1979). If these important findings are confirmed it will be possible not only to transfer many children from the functional, presumed psychogenic, category to the organic

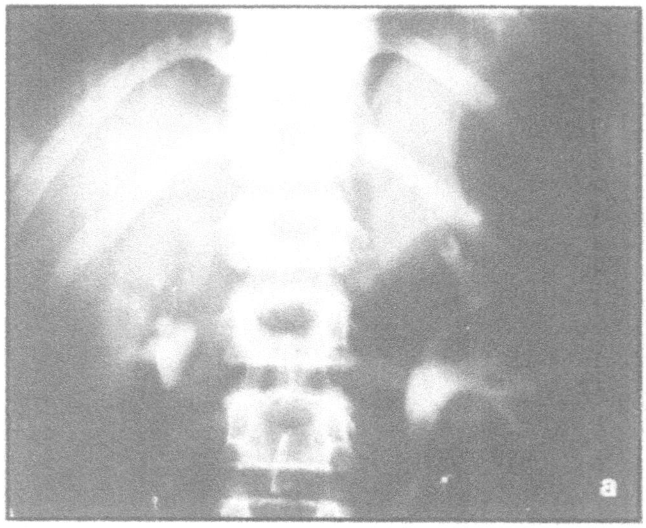

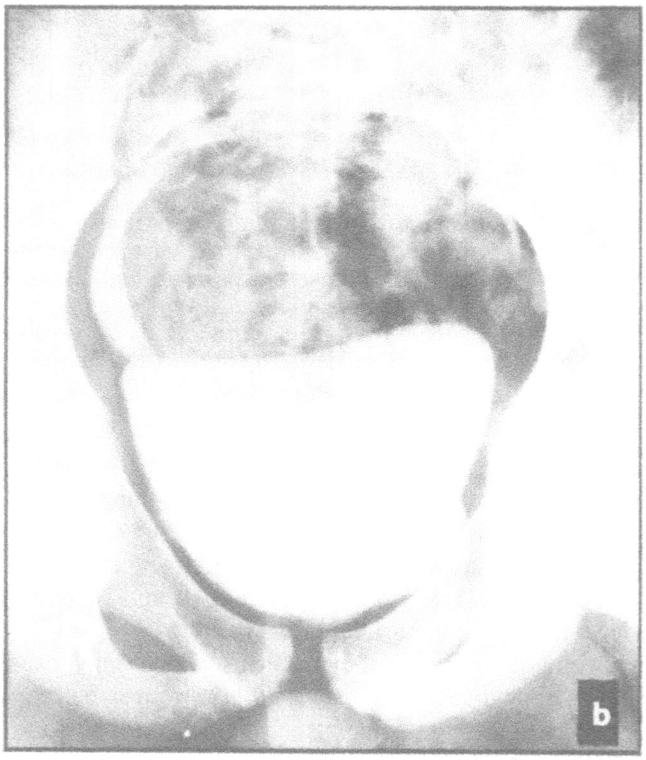

Figure 12.5. *a) The IVU and b) the cystogram of a 12-year-old boy who presented with long-standing, right-sided abdominal pain. The right kidney is small and there is right ureteric reflux. His pain was abolished by right ureteric reimplantation.*

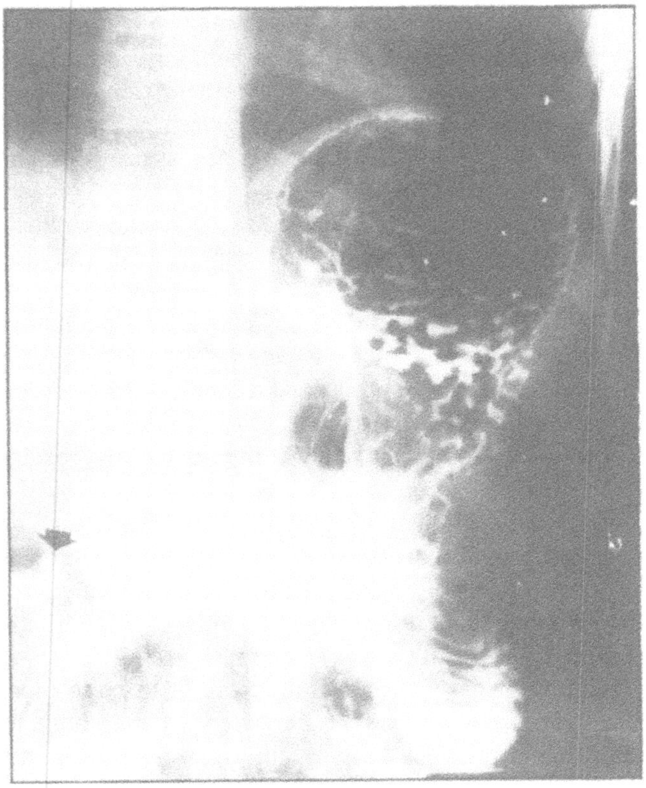

Figure 12.6. *The barium meal of an eight-year-old boy who presented with epigastric pain. Coarse gastric mucosal folds and an ulcer crater (arrowed) are shown.*

category but also to offer a safe and effective method of dietary treatment. A therapeutic trial of milk exclusion in children with unexplained recurrent pain certainly seems worthwhile.

'Functional' Abdominal Pain

The features of 'functional' abdominal pain are variable. The onset may be at any time in childhood but there are peaks at around five years and at puberty. In about two-thirds the pain is confined to the umbilical region but radiation to one side or the other and pain in the epigastric region as well as centrally occurs quite frequently. A constant aching pain is described slightly more often than intermittent colicky spasms. Although half the children have only mild pain, in many it is moderate and in some severe. Regular periodicity of the pain is unusual. Associated symptoms are common, nausea and/or pallor occur in about half, and headache, vomiting and/or sleepiness in about one quarter of the patients. Compared with controls, the families of affected children show a much higher incidence of abdominal pain and a significant increase in peptic ulceration, appendicectomy, migraine and nervous breakdown.

Pathogenic Mechanisms

Some possible pathogenic mechanisms are listed in Table 12.2. In the majority of children the primary mechanisms seem likely to be psychogenic. Occasional abdominal discomfort is a universal experience and most, perhaps all, children at some time discover the pleasing effects which can be achieved by adding an element of histrionic exaggeration. Sensible parents recognize this experiment for what it is and avoid offering too positive a response for fear of perpetuating the behaviour pattern. What could be more delightful, and more positively reinforcing, than universal sympathy and concern, a day off school, a pleasant-tasting potion, a light but appetizing diet and a warm bed? Less sensible parents often have cause to regret their well-intentioned overconcern and eventually resort to the doctor for assistance in extricating themselves from this trap of their own making. The strong familial tendency to develop such symptoms may result from an inherited predisposition as well as a learned response. It seems probable that in many children both these factors play a part.

In some children the symptoms are very similar to those of so-called spastic colon in adults and the two conditions, and possibly also infantile colic, may be analogous. Constipation is certainly a cause of recurrent pain in some children and is usually apparent from the history and the findings of large indentable masses in the colon and hard faeces in the dilated rectum. We are impressed that air swallowing is another cause of significant pain in some children. The girl whose radiograph is shown in Figure 12.7 has had recurrent bouts of pain and pseudo-obstruction. Like most such children, if closely observed she could be seen gulping air. Recurrent dietary indiscretions can obviously be a cause of pain. Finally, there is an excess of little bellyachers in families prone to migraine and it seems reasonable to suppose that similar mechanisms may be involved.

Clinical Management

The clinical management of the child with functional abdominal pain and his family is an exercise more in the art than the science of medicine. By the time the doctor

Table 12.2. 'Functional' causes of recurrent abdominal pain.

Psychogenic/behaviour problem
Spastic colon
Constipation
Air-swallowing
Dietary indiscretions
Periodic syndrome/migraine equivalent

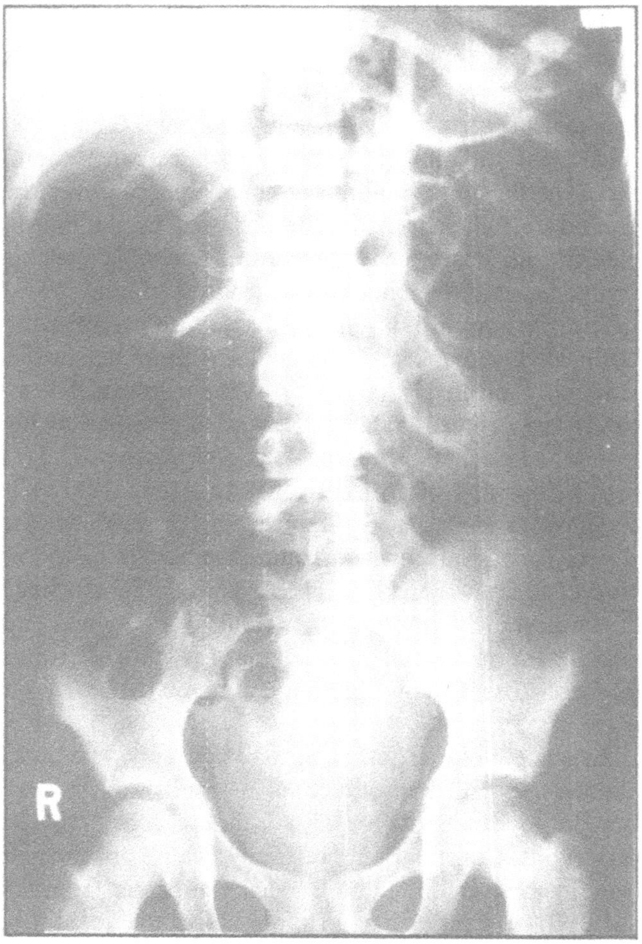

Figure 12.7. *Gross gaseous intestinal distension in a 10-year-old girl who presented with recurrent abdominal pain due to swallowing of air.*

is consulted a considerable amount of anxiety has usually built up and its dissipation may be dramatically therapeutic. The first essential, as emphasized above, is a demonstrably full and careful history and examination with specific consideration and exclusion of organic disease. Apart from the obligatory urine test we would recommend investigations only as indicated even though we are aware of the therapeutic power of a diagnostic x-ray and blood test!

When organic disease has been excluded, and has been seen to be excluded, careful explanation and reassurance is needed. We like to lay special emphasis on three points. First, a thorough clinical evaluation has revealed no sign of organic illness. It is often helpful to exclude by name conditions which may be feared, such as appendicitis, intra-abdominal tumours, bowel obstruction and leukaemia. It is worth learning of any particular fear which may be harboured in the family and excluding it, using appropriate special investigations if necessary.

Second, it is important to explain that, although there is no demonstrable cause, the pain is real and not imagined or feigned.

Third, the fact that abdominal pain is a very common stress response in children is emphasized. The concept of stress-induced symptoms and a family predisposition to headaches, abdominal pain, skin problems or some other common psychogenic entity is usually readily accepted.

Unless there is a specific treatable problem, such as constipation, drug treatment has little to offer, although sedatives, analgesics, antispasmodics, anticholinergics, psychotropics and others have been advocated. Perhaps a placebo should always be given first!

If underlying environmental stress factors are present, consideration should be given to measures to correct the problem by separating the child from the bullying peer, the classroom martinet, the amorous uncle or other avoidable social hazard. If the child is more deeply disturbed, psychotherapy has a place in management but, fortunately for the overstretched services, this is the exception rather than the rule.

Follow-up Studies

Follow-up studies by Apley and others indicated that, for children whose problem was sufficiently severe to warrant referral to hospital, the prognosis was rather disappointing. In adult life, approximately one third were free from symptoms, one third continued to have abdominal pain and one third had other problems, such as migraine or neurotic symptoms. This is, therefore, by no means a trivial matter and one well worthy of our time and trouble—even at the end of that long surgery!

References

Apley, J., *The Child with Abdominal Pains* (2nd edition), Blackwell Scientific Publications, London, 1975.

Barr, R. G., Levine, M. D. and Watkins, J. B., *New Engl. J. Med.*, 1979, **300**, 1449.

Jackson, R. H., *Br. Med. J.*, 1963, **2**, 277.

13. Pyrexia of Unknown Origin

FEVER is the commonest single presenting sign of illness in childhood. In this chapter we will discuss the diagnostic approach to children with fever of unknown origin, that is, fever for which the cause is not apparent from the history and clinical examination. This is, of course, a daily dilemma for general practitioners and paediatricians.

Temperature Recording

First, some general points on temperature recording. In spite of the universal availability of and familiarity with clinical thermometers, accurate recording of the temperature in the home is seldom achieved. Often it is reported simply that the child was flushed or felt hot, and yet the presence or absence of fever and its type and degree may be important considerations in differential diagnosis.

The axillary temperature is difficult to record accurately and is usually 0.5°C lower than the oral temperature, which is in turn 0.5°C lower than the rectal, oesophageal, or aural temperature which reflect most accurately the core temperature. When taking the axillary temperature the thermometer should be left in situ for at least one minute and ideally reinserted for a further 30 seconds after removal to ensure that no further rise occurs. When taking the oral temperature a similar time is necessary for equilibration. To record the rectal temperature in an infant it is important to insert the (lubricated) end of the thermometer for a distance of at least 2 to 2.5 cm to obtain an accurate measurement of core temperature.

The oral temperature will, of course, be affected by hot or cold food or drink recently ingested. Exercise, including vigorous crying or a prolonged fit, will cause a rise in body temperature, especially in a hot environment.

The mean normal temperature is 37°C (98.4°F). Normal children, especially if they have been active, may have a temperature about 0.5°C above this value during the afternoon or early evening. This is sometimes documented by anxious parents, who produce carefully plotted temperature charts. This degree of temperature variation may simply represent normal circadian rhythm. Such children were aptly called 'ninety-niners' by Dr Douglas Gairdner. Their parents should be encouraged to lock the thermometer away and to use it only after consultation with their physician!

Pyrexias of Known Origin

We will not discuss those febrile illnesses, the great majority, accompanied by symptoms or signs which permit a provisional diagnosis to be made. Fever itself may, of course, be associated with nonspecific symptoms such as malaise, headache, anorexia and myalgia. In infants many conditions may present as PUO which, in older children and adults, would pose no diagnostic problem because of the history. Physical examination also poses more difficulties but we will assume that relatively subtle signs, such as an inflamed eardrum or Koplik's spots, are never missed!

Fever of Acute Onset in Children Previously Well

Bacterial Septicaemia

The most difficult task is to identify the child who is seriously ill. The course of bacterial septicaemia, for instance that caused by the meningococcus, may be extremely rapid and the outlook is entirely dependent upon the stage at which appropriate treatment is started. Definite signs, such as petechiae, cyanosis or peripheral vascular collapse will not be disregarded, but sometimes the general practitioner must rely on his clinical sixth sense to pick out the few really ill children from the many with minor illness. If that sixth sense is alerted, even in the absence of objective findings, the safest course is to admit the child to hospital for observation but, if he is to remain at home, he must be seen again within a very few hours. Careful examination of the naked child in a good light is essential to detect the earliest appearance of the tell-tale rash (Figure 13.1).

Meningitis and Encephalitis

Infection of the central nervous system is frequently associated with septicaemia. It is often easy to diagnose because of obvious meningism, focal fits or other definite findings, but many features of the illness, such as clouding of the sensorium, headache and photophobia, are nonspecific. Signs of meningism may be difficult or impossible to elicit in the infant under two years of age especially when he is irritable and fractious. It is important to remember that meningitis may present with a febrile convulsion. Children with partially treated meningitis (Figure 13.2) and tuberculous meningitis present particularly difficult diagnostic problems. Every child in whom there is a suspicion of meningitis must have a lumbar puncture. Procrastination in this situation may prove disastrous and all children's departments are prepared to admit children briefly to exclude meningitis. If the cerebrospinal fluid proves to be clear the child can often be allowed home.

Urinary Tract Infection (UTI)

In older children UTI usually presents with dysuria and frequency with or without signs of upper tract involvement, such as loin pain. Secondary nocturnal enuresis is another useful clue to infection. However, in children under two years of age, UTI frequently presents as PUO. A bag or 'clean-catch' urine specimen must therefore be examined in all infants without an obvious cause for their fever. In this way cases of UTI associated with renal tract malformation, such as ureteric reflux, may be detected before progressive renal damage

Figure 13.1. *An infant showing the faint petechial rash of early meningococcal septicaemia. (For the established rash, see figure 15.3, page 109.)*

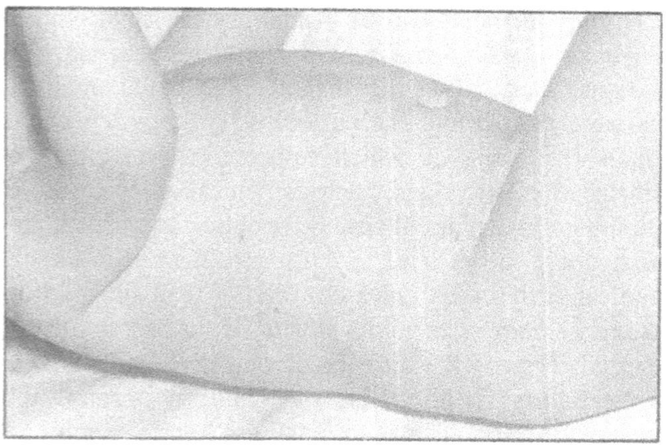

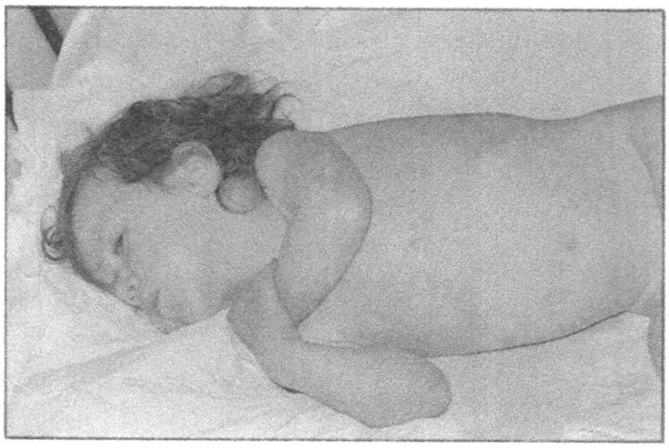

Figure 13.1. *An infant showing the faint petechial rash of early meningococcal septicaemia. (For the established rash, see figure 15.3, page 109.)*

occurs. Proven UTI in a preschool child of either sex should be an absolute indication for an intravenous pyelogram and a micturating cystourethrogram (see chapter 10).

Bone and Joint Infection

Bone and joint infections may present as PUO, especially in infants. Painstaking and methodical examination is needed to identify the bone or joint affected. This is another problem for which hospital management is essential. Investigation may require isotopic imaging and surgery as well as repeated blood cultures.

Tropical Diseases

A history of recent foreign travel is usually the clue that PUO is due to tropical disease, which may present after the patient's return home. Malaria and typhoid must be considered, as well as typhus, dengue, other parasitic infections and Lassa fever. Specialist help will often be necessary in the definitive diagnosis of these conditions.

Viral Infections

These are by far the commonest causes of PUO. They may be subdivided into nonspecific and specific viral infections.

Nonspecific Infections

Infants and children may have as many as six to ten minor infections annually. In most of these episodes, symptoms of upper or lower respiratory tract infection will be present but often there is a total lack of clinical findings other than fever and misery. As long as the general practitioner is confident that no serious condition is present, observation with symptomatic treatment at home is usually appropriate.

Specific Infections

In the incubation period of many viral illnesses, such as the common exanthemata, there may be fever without other findings, but the culprit shortly declares itself. Other important conditions include the following:

Roseola infantum (exanthema subitum, sixth disease). This common illness may cause considerable anxiety. The patient, usually an infant, has a high and unremitting fever for three or four days but seems reasonably well and on examination is otherwise normal. The temperature then falls suddenly and the child is covered in a generalized morbilliform rash which rapidly resolves. One clinical clue during the pyrexial phase is the characteristically low polymorphonuclear count.

Anicteric hepatitis A. Affected children are listless, anorexic and only mildly febrile. Excess urobilinogen can be detected in the urine and the diagnosis confirmed by liver enzyme studies. It is important to detect this disease for epidemiological reasons.

Glandular fever. Infection with the Epstein-Barr virus may cause only fever and malaise although more commonly lymphadenopathy, an infected throat (see figure 4.4, page 36), enlargement of the spleen or a rash may be found. If broad spectrum antibiotics of the ampicillin group are prescribed, a generalized maculopapular rash almost invariably develops (Figure 13.3). The diagnosis can be made by demonstration of atypical mononuclear cells in the blood film, a positive Paul-Bunnell test or a positive Epstein-Barr virus complement fixation test. Glandular fever is rare under the age of six years. It may occasionally be mimicked by cytomegalovirus infection and toxoplasmosis.

Mycoplasma Infection

Disease due to *Mycoplasma* is especially common in children of school age and may present with fever and nonspecific upper respiratory tract symptoms only. Characteristically, the chest x-ray appearances of consolidation are more impressive than the symptoms and physical findings would suggest (see figure 5.7, page 45). The diagnosis may be confirmed by demonstration of cold agglutinins and the specific complement fixation test.

Fever in the Newborn

Fever (and also hypothermia) in the newborn infant may be an important sign of serious illness, and septicaemia, meningitis and urinary tract infection especially

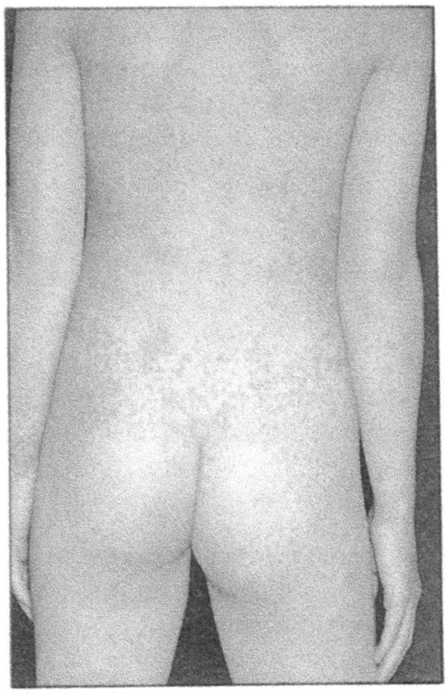

Figure 13.3. *Morbilliform rash in a boy with glandular fever who was given ampicillin.*

require exclusion. There are, however, three benign pyrexial states which should be mentioned: maternal fever, the overheated baby and dehydration fever.

Maternal Fever

The fetal temperature is 0.5°C higher than the maternal temperature. The infant of a mother with fever may have a raised temperature for several hours after birth. No treatment is required, but the infant may need special supervision because of his exposure to the condition responsible for the maternal fever.

The Overheated Baby

It is very easy to overheat newborn babies inadvertently by injudicious use of swaddling, incubators, radiant heat shields and phototherapy units or by exposure to a high temperature from heating units or sunlight. If the infant is otherwise well it is reasonable to place him in a more appropriate thermal environment in the expectation that his temperature will return to normal over the following few hours.

Dehydration Fever

If for any reason, the most common being inadequately established breast feeding, a newborn baby loses more than 10 per cent of his body weight, he may develop fever. Dehydration will be apparent and the serum osmolality will be in excess of 300 mOsm/kg H_2O. Rehydration is associated with a prompt decline in the fever. This syndrome may occasionally be seen with water-losing states, such as diabetes insipidus, in older children.

PUO in Children Especially at Risk of Infection

Fever in children especially at risk requires prompt and full evaluation, usually in hospital. Although the total number of such children is small, a considerable proportion of the diagnostically difficult and confusing episodes of feverish illness occurs among them. The more important categories include the following:

Children with prostheses in contact with the circulation. Such children have had either neurosurgical, most frequently ventriculoatrial shunting, or cardiac surgical procedures. Any episode of PUO must be considered to be due to bacterial colonization of the prosthesis until proven otherwise. The infection may be with organisms of low virulence and the diagnosis may be difficult to prove, sometimes requiring special measures such as aspiration of a shunt. A complication of such disease is immune-complex nephritis. Correct treatment will depend both on the bacteriological diagnosis and consideration of the associated plumbing problem.

Children with congenital heart disease. Children with a ventricular septal defect, patent ductus arteriosus and congenital valvular lesions are particularly at risk from subacute bacterial endocarditis. They must, of course, have antibiotic prophylaxis for all dental procedures and for any other surgery which may result in transient bacteraemia (see chapter 9). SBE should always be considered first in children with fever and CHD but suspicion will be particularly high in the presence of altered cardiac signs, such as heart failure, embolic phenomena, splenomegaly or tachycardia out of proportion to the fever. Multiple blood cultures may be necessary for confirmation of the diagnosis.

Children after splenectomy. Surgical removal of the spleen, and also congenital absence of the organ or loss of function from infarction in sickle cell anaemia, is associated with an increased incidence of fulminant septicaemic illness, most frequently due to the pneumococcus. The danger is greater the younger the child when the spleen was removed and the more severe the problem necessitating the splenectomy. The risk is small after splenectomy for traumatic rupture of the spleen, greater in patients with spherocytosis or portal hypertension, and greater still in those with reticulosis or thalassaemia. PUO in such children is an urgent indication for blood culture and therapy with intravenous penicillin, and indeed, most paediatricians prefer to maintain them on continuous prophylactic penicillin. They should be given Pneumovax (see chapter 2).

Immunodeficiency and immunosuppression. This group includes children with primary or secondary immunodeficiency states, those receiving immunosuppressive agents or radiotherapy for leukaemia or malignant disease, and children on steroids or other immunosuppressive drugs for other reasons. Such children are particularly at risk from unusual infective agents, such as fungi and protozoa, and they require full and prompt investigation for any obscure febrile illness.

Less Common Causes of PUO in Childhood

Children with these conditions tend to show a more chronic disease pattern, and in addition to fever they are likely to have anorexia, weight loss, depression and ill-localized aches and pains. Table 13.1 lists the final diagnoses reached in a series of 100 children with PUO who presented with fever greater than 38.5°C persisting for more than two weeks (Pizzo et al. 1975). It is interesting to note how many of these conditions could presumably have been diagnosed clinically at an earlier stage. Any child with a prolonged feverish illness warrants repeated thorough physical examination. We will briefly consider some of the more important conditions which may present in this way.

Table 13.1. Final diagnosis in 100 children with fever persisting for more than two weeks (Pizzo et al. 1975, with permission).

Infections 53	
17 Viral, nonspecific	3 Endocarditis
5 Tonsillitis	2 Glandular fever
4 UTI	2 Osteomyelitis
4 Pneumonia	2 Typhoid
4 Septicaemia	1 Generalized herpes
3 Meningitis	1 Malaria
3 Sinusitis	1 Tuberculosis
	1 Hepatitis
Collagen Disease 13	
10 Rheumatoid arthritis	
3 Systemic lupus erythematosus	
Malignancy 6	
4 Leukaemia	
2 Lymphoma	
Gastrointestinal 6	
4 Crohn's disease	
1 Ulcerative colitis	
1 Ruptured appendix	
Miscellaneous 10	
Undiagnosed 12	

Infectious Diseases

Infectious diseases that cause prolonged feverish illnesses are summarized in Table 13.2.

Rheumatic Fever

Although now a rare condition, rheumatic fever should not be forgotten. The diagnosis rests on evidence of current or recent streptococcal infection associated with other manifestations, including fever, carditis, polyarthritis, erythema marginatum, subcutaneous nodules and chorea.

Still's Disease

The child with Still's disease may present with a high swinging fever for some weeks before other stigmata, such as arthritis, iritis or a skin rash appear (Figure 13.4). Such patients are seronegative and, apart from nonspecific acute phase protein changes, such as a raised ESR and increased alpha-2 globulin, blood tests are unhelpful. Occasionally, after other causes of fever have been excluded, a diagnostic and therapeutic trial of steroids may be necessary, the child with Still's disease showing a dramatic response.

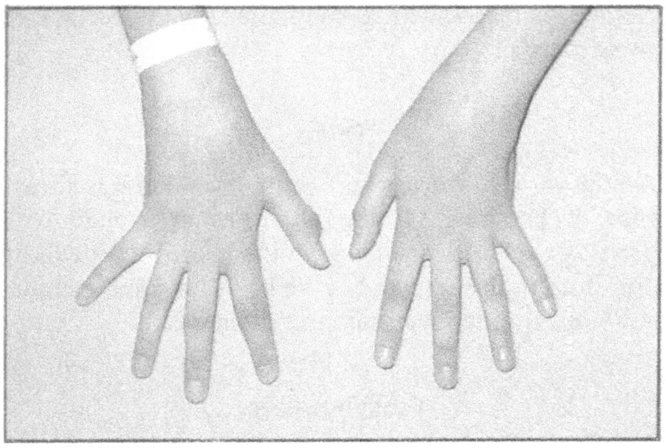

Figure 13.4. *Arthritis of the wrists and some finger joints in a girl with Still's disease who initially presented with PUO.*

Collagen Diseases

This group of conditions is rare in childhood and yet more rarely presents as PUO since there are usually other obvious manifestations, such as skin lesions, arthritis, renal or haematological problems with characteristic serological evidence of disordered immune processes.

Malignant Disease

Fortunately, malignant disease is a much less common cause of PUO in childhood than in adult life. However, leukaemia, Hodgkin's disease and other lymphomas and solid tumours can present in this way.

Crohn's Disease

Crohn's disease must be considered in the chronically ill child with fever and vague gastrointestinal symptoms.

Inadequate Heat Loss

In feverish infants, marked peripheral vasoconstriction may develop, especially when vigorous cooling methods, such as cold sponging and fanning, are used. The effect will be exaggerated when there is peripheral vascular shut-down due to fluid loss. Such infants are unable to lose heat at an adequate rate and so characteristically have a high core temperature and relatively low skin temperature. Expansion of the intravascular fluid volume with blood or plasma and, if necessary, the use of alpha-blocking drugs in small doses, will restore proper equilibrium. A similar problem may occur in

Table 13.2. Less common infective causes of PUO in childhood.

Disease	Clinical clues	Confirmatory tests
Local abscess formation (brain, dental, pulmonary, subphrenic, etc.)	Preceding illness with partial resolution, leucocytosis	X-rays, isotopic scans
Tuberculosis	Immigrant contact	Tuberculin test, chest x-ray
Myocarditis, pericarditis	Tachycardia, chest pain	ECG, Coxsackie virus titres
Typhoid, other salmonellosis	Foreign travel, cough, GI symptoms	Blood, stool culture, Widal test
Brucellosis	Foreign travel or rural domicile, contact with farm animals, unpasteurized milk	Blood culture, antibody titre
Cat scratch fever	Contact with cats	Skin test, gland histology
Q fever	Respiratory symptoms	Coxiella antibody titre

children with ectodermal dysplasia because of lack of sweat glands.

Drugs

A wide variety of drugs may cause fever and it is always wise, if possible, to stop all drugs in a child with persistent PUO. Sulphonamides are particularly notorious in this respect but the list is long and includes antibiotics, anticonvulsants and analgesics.

Factitious Fever

The possibility of malingering must not be forgotten. Fever with a normal pulse rate and a lack of other symptoms, especially in an adolescent with psychological disturbance, may arouse suspicion. Taking the temperature under close supervision may solve the problem and it has also been suggested that measurement of urinary temperature with a fast-reading electronic thermometer could be useful.

Exotica

Some rare causes of PUO in childhood are listed in Table 13.3.

Table 13.3. Rare causes of PUO in childhood.

Periodic syndrome
Appendicitis
CNS disease, including subdural haematoma, hypothalamic disorder
Familial dysautonomia (Riley-Day syndrome)
Familial Mediterranean fever
Sarcoidosis
Cholangitis, liver disease
Infantile cortical hyperostosis (Caffey's disease)

Investigation of PUO

In Table 13.4 we have tried to summarize appropriate investigations at home and in hospital. In most cases the clinical findings and first line investigations will indicate which channels should be more thoroughly explored. In many situations the crucial investigation is the blood culture and repeated cultures should be made.

Table 13.4. Investigation of PUO.

Investigation at home
Urinalysis and culture
Full blood count, ESR
Nose swab, throat swab, stool culture
Monospot, Paul-Bunnell
Tuberculin test
Chest x-ray
Further investigation in hospital
Blood cultures
Serum proteins, immunoglobulins
Serological tests for specific bacteria, viruses
LE cells, antinuclear factor, complement levels, etc.
ECG
CSF examination, culture
IVP, skeletal survey, barium studies, angiography, etc.
Isotopic scans, liver, bone, etc.
Bone marrow examination, culture, blood smears
Organ biopsy, gland biopsy, laparotomy

Management

It is vitally important in PUO to avoid blind antibiotic therapy before a microbiological diagnosis has been made, except in the critically ill child, to whom, after appropriate cultures have been obtained, antibiotics can be administered intravenously in combinations designed to combat all organisms, both aerobic and anaerobic, which might underlie the illness. Hospital admission is, of course, necessary in this situation.

Fever can generally be controlled with simple antipyretics such as aspirin or paracetamol. If this proves insufficient, tepid sponging can also be used. Control of the fever is particularly important in infants, especially those known to be at risk of febrile convulsions.

It can be difficult to decide whether a child with PUO should be managed at home or referred to hospital and the decision will, of course, rest largely on the general practitioner's assessment of the severity of the illness. As a general principle, however, it seems wise not to allow fever to persist for more than about a week before making strenuous efforts to elucidate the cause.

Reference

Pizzo, P. A., Lovejoy, F. H. and Smith, D. H., *Pediatrics,* 1975, **55**, 468.

14. Diabetes Mellitus

DIABETES is uncommon in childhood, approximately one child in 800 under the age of 16 being affected. A general practitioner with an average list can therefore expect to have only one diabetic child among his flock. This particular lamb, however, may well cause more than his fair share of trouble and anxiety to the shepherd!

For practical purposes diabetes in childhood is always of the juvenile-onset, ketosis-prone type now known as type 1. Other types, such as maturity-onset diabetes of the young, glucose intolerance complicating inherited syndromes and iatrogenic diabetes, usually from steroid therapy, are rare and, although of theoretical interest, will not be considered further.

Aetiology

It is likely that three chief factors are important in the pathogenesis of juvenile-onset diabetes: a genetic predisposition, a viral trigger and an autoimmune mechanism (see Farquhar 1979). The evidence for a genetic predisposition is derived from the familial but non-mendelian pattern of the disease, the identical twin studies which show a considerable degree of concordance (although, perhaps surprisingly, considerably less than for maturity-onset diabetes which has a larger genetic component) and over-representation of certain HL-A groups, notably DR3, DR4, A8 and W15. Indications that a viral trigger may initiate the disease include epidemiological clues, such as the increased frequency of presentation in the winter months and in the first years at school, and more direct evidence incriminating certain viruses, such as mumps, Coxsackie B and congenital rubella in rare cases. A high incidence of islet cell and other antibodies can be demonstrated in juvenile diabetes of recent onset, and it is plausible to postulate that a self-destructive mechanism may cause the gradual and progressive loss of islet cell function which characterizes juvenile diabetes in the months after presentation.

Presentation

Polyuria and polydipsia are the cardinal symptoms of juvenile diabetes. At presentation about 50 per cent of children will have had these symptoms for between three and six weeks, 25 per cent for a shorter, and 25 per cent for a longer time. Untreated, the child develops ketoacidosis with a ketotic odour to the breath (ability to detect the characteristic 'pear-drop' smell varies greatly) and deep, sighing acidotic breathing. Eventually there is progressive clouding of consciousness followed by deep coma and death.

Delay in diagnosis may occur when the parents, and occasionally the doctor, dismiss the early symptoms as being due to the weather, habit, a behaviour problem or cystitis. Diagnostic confusion may also arise when the polyuria and polydipsia are overshadowed by other symptoms, notably those of localized infection, weight loss, polyphagia or anorexia, vomiting or abdominal pain. It is therefore essential to test the urine of all children with acute abdominal pain for this among other reasons (see chapter 12).

Management

We will not consider the treatment of ketoacidosis, an acute medical emergency, or the initial stabilization of the diabetic child, which is best undertaken in hospital unless exceptional home care facilities are available.

The main aim of all the members of the medical team should be to render themselves redundant as soon as possible! However conscientious and available they may be, they can provide advice only on coarse adjustment of the diabetic regime; hour-to-hour and day-to-day decisions on fine adjustment must be made by the child and/or his parents and good control can never be achieved unless they have clear understanding of the basic principles of management. As the diabetic child grows up, he must become independent not only of his doctors but also of his parents. We strongly encourage children to take over responsibility for their injections and urine testing from the age of eight years at the latest. The activities of the British Diabetic Association, especially their organized summer camps, are of inestimable value in helping children to become independent and in relieving them from the sense of isolation which the rarity of the disease often engenders.

The essential concept to emphasize in teaching a diabetic child is, of course, the control of blood glucose by insulin. Once this is thoroughly grasped it is relatively simple to consider the effect on this balance of other factors, such as exertion, emotion, illness, residual insulin secretion and the details of an insulin and dietary regime. It is essential also for the child to be fully conversant with the details of injection technique, urine testing and, ideally, home blood glucose monitoring.

We will consider briefly the three major elements of the diabetic management regime, diet, insulin and exertion.

Diet

Regularity, not restriction, is the key to a satisfactory diet for the juvenile diabetic. Some degree of carbohydrate control is essential and the carbohydrate content of the diet, preferably not given in highly refined and rapidly absorbed form, should be evenly spread through the day in the main meals and between-meal snacks. For example, 25 per cent of total carbohydrate content for breakfast, 10 per cent for mid-morning snack, 25 per cent for lunch, 10 per cent for mid-afternoon snack, 25 per cent for supper and 5 per cent before bed would be suitable. Such a schedule of almost continuous eating is fortunately well suited to most children and most insulin regimes! There is no need to reduce the total carbohydrate content of the diet unless the child is overweight; indeed, it is probably desirable for approximately 60 per cent of total calories to be derived from carbohydrate rather than the 40 per cent of the average English diet. This results in improved diabetic control and a lower intake of fat, which is desirable as diabetics are atheroma-prone. A generous intake of unabsorbed fibre and an increased ratio of polyunsaturated to saturated fat are also advised. Although compromises must always be made, most diabetic children accept a diet based on these principles and stray from it no more and no less than expected!

Insulin

Many changes are in progress in insulin manufacture and methods of delivery but to date these have had only a limited impact on the management of juvenile diabetes. This remains based on once- or twice-daily subcutaneous injection of sustained action or mixed short and sustained action insulin preparations. A majority of prepubertal and a minority of pubertal children can maintain good blood glucose control on a single daily injection, but many diabetologists prefer routinely to use two injections because of the greater flexibility and adaptability this offers. It is our practice to use a once-daily regime only in those children in whom good control is easily achieved.

There is a confusing plethora of new insulin preparations on the market as all manufacturers follow the lead of the Scandinavians in producing highly purified preparations. These are less antigenic than the old 'dirty' preparations but their only definite short-term advantage is freedom from the previously common and distressing side-effect of fat atrophy (Figure 14.1). However, since there is at least a theoretical possibility that their long-term use may be associated with less rapid development of microvascular and macrovascular diabetic complications, it seems prudent for all diabetic children to have them. Porcine insulin also has a theoretical advantage over the bovine product since the insulin molecule is more similar to that of human insulin.

Our currently preferred regimes are once-daily Actrapid and Monotard or twice-daily Velosulin and Insulatard since these were the first highly purified insulins to become available but many other regimes are equally satisfactory. Some details of insulins suitable

Figure 14.1. *The arm of a diabetic child showing lipoatrophy at an insulin injection site.*

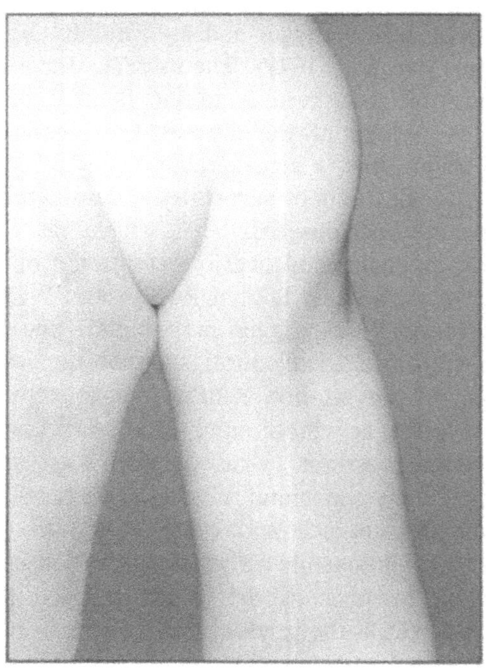

Table 14.1. Highly purified insulins suitable for use in diabetic children.

	Type	Source	Approx. duration of action by subcutaneous injection (hours)		
			Onset	Maximum	Finish
Short-acting:					
Actrapid Velosulin Hypurin Neutral Neusulin	Neutral soluble	Pig Pig Cow Cow	½	2-4	8
Intermediate-acting:					
Insulatard Hypurin Isophane Neuphane	Isophane	Pig Cow Cow	2	6-12	24
Monotard	Zinc suspension lente	Pig			

for use in children are shown in Table 14.1. Although a number of ready mixed preparations are available, we prefer not to use these, except in special circumstances, because of their lack of flexibility.

It is useful to remember that average daily insulin requirements in the preadolescent are approximately 0.75 to 1.0 units/kg/day and in the adolescent 1.0 to 1.5 units/kg/day.

Exertion

Physical activity has a potent insulin-like effect on the blood glucose. Regularity is therefore, once again, the key to this important aspect of the diabetic's life. We encourage regular exercise both for its well known effect on the moral fibre and for its effect on the cardiovascular system! Unfortunately, regularity is seldom achieved in childhood: school-age children often play games or do long, cross-country runs only once or twice a week, and teenagers tend to loll about all day and then dance the night away in discos. Such irregular exertions are best allowed for by taking extra carbohydrate beforehand, 10 to 20 g covering most activities. If more consistent exertion is planned, as on an active holiday, adjustment of the insulin or dietary regime may be necessary.

Assessment of Control

The aim of the treatment of juvenile diabetes is to maintain the blood glucose within the normal range for as much of the time as possible consistent with living an active and relatively unrestricted life. Present evidence suggests that if normoglycaemia is achieved the secondary metabolic effects and complications of the disease are prevented. The most useful clinical indicators of control are growth and development, routine urine tests, timed urine collections, home blood glucose monitoring and haemoglobin A_1 tests.

Growth and Development

Severe diabetic imbalance results in acute symptoms from hypoglycaemia or ketosis, but normal growth and development is a sensitive indicator of adequate control over the longer term. The poorly controlled diabetic child falls further and further from his previous growth channel; his bone age lags behind his chronological age and his pubertal development is delayed; he may develop hepatomegaly and other diabetic complications, such as necrobiosis lipoidica diabeticorum (Figure 14.2).

Routine Urine Tests

These remain the cornerstone of day-to-day assessment of control for most juvenile diabetics. The 2-drop Clinitest method, which records up to 5 per cent glycosuria, is more useful for children than the 5-drop method. Suitable instructions and colour charts can be obtained from the manufacturers, Ames Ltd (Figure 14.3). The most useful urine specimens are second voidings before breakfast, before the main meals and at bedtime, but it is obviously unrealistic to expect children to perform such a complicated ritual four times daily for a long period. The number and timing of the tests requested must therefore strike a compromise between the ideal and the possible. Even so, many of the urine testing charts brought to diabetic clinics owe their existence entirely to the imagination. This is often obvious when, for instance, the recordings spill into the days yet to come, but may be misleading when more care has been taken with presentation! Some children who refuse to test their urine with Clinitest tablets are

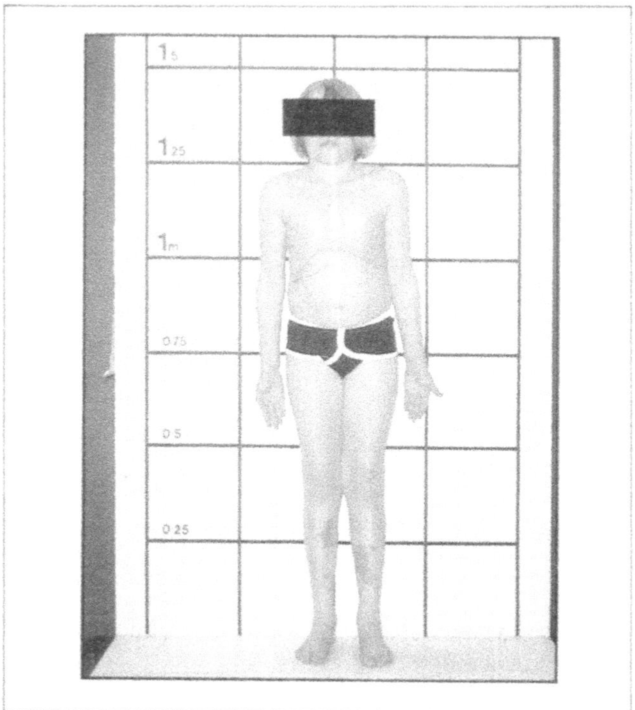

Figure 14.2. *A 15-year-old diabetic boy showing grossly retarded growth, moderate liver enlargement (marked) and necrobiosis lipoidica diabeticorum on his shins, all consequent upon poor diabetic control.*

willing to use the simpler but rather less accurate Diastix or Testape methods. Ideally, the majority of urine tests will be negative and only occasional samples will show heavy glycosuria.

Timed Urine Collections

Total 24-hour urine glucose loss provides a useful objective method of assessing control. Good control can be defined as a loss of less than 10 per cent of the dietary carbohydrate content in the urine as glucose. Timed collection for periods less than 24 hours can be extremely helpful in elucidating, for example, escape from control through the night hours or for a certain part of the day, and can be of real help in adjusting the insulin or dietary regime. Most laboratories are willing to measure the glucose content of timed urine collections, and approximate, but clinically useful, estimations can be achieved at home by measuring the volume of urine passed in a specified time period and the concentration of glucose with Clinitest.

Figure 14.3. *Clinitest 2-drop method, urine testing instructions and colour chart.*

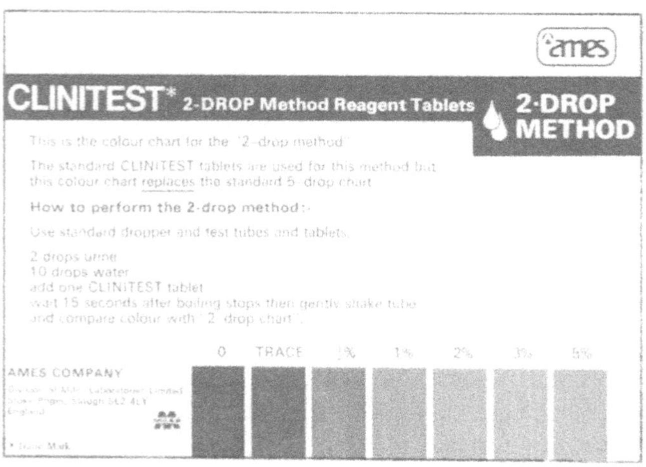

Home Blood Glucose Monitoring

The availability of Dextrostix testing strips and reflectance meters[1] has brought accurate blood glucose measurement at home within the competence and the pocket of most families with diabetic children. This method of assessment proved unacceptable to many children until the development of mechanical finger-prickers enabled an adequate drop of blood to be obtained simply and almost entirely painlessly. (In our experience much the most satisfactory device is the Autolet[2].) Using this apparatus most diabetic children will accept multiple daily finger-pricks for prolonged periods and many express strong preference for this method over urine testing. It offers, of course, the major additional advantage that the blood glucose can be maintained within the physiological range. It is especially useful when reliable urine testing is difficult, as in very young children and those with low renal thresholds. We now teach this method routinely and recommend it whenever appropriate.

Haemoglobin A_1

This test measures the amount of glycosylated haemoglobin present in the blood, which is proportional to the mean blood glucose over the life of the red cell. It thus provides an objective indication of the adequacy of diabetic control for the previous two months or so, and it has proved the answer to one of the most frequent prayers of the paediatric diabetologist! Its early promise has been fulfilled and it is generally accepted to be the most useful indication of diabetic control in the medium term. The norms vary according to the laboratory and the method of estimation used but this test should be

[1] Currently we favour the Hypocount, available from Hypoguard Ltd, 49 Grimston Lane, Trimley, Ipswich, Suffolk IP10 0SA and the Glucometer, available from Ames Co Ltd, PO Box 37, Stoke Court, Stoke Poges, Slough, Berks SL2 4LY.

[2] Autolet can be obtained from Owen Mumford Ltd, Medical Division, Brook Hill, Woodstock, Oxon OX7 1TU.

available for the assessment of all juvenile diabetics. We regularly receive both good and bad surprises when HbA_1 estimations conflict with our assessment of control by less objective methods.

Problems in Management

Most problems in the management of juvenile diabetes centre around difficulty in maintaining good control of the blood glucose. It is often stated that children have more 'brittle' diabetes than adults but, in fact, intrinsically unstable diabetes is rare in children and it is the nature of the beast rather than the disease that is brittle! The more frequent reasons for difficulty with control can be considered broadly as either failures of compliance or failures of comprehension.

Failures of Compliance

Overt failure to comply with treatment is simple to detect but difficult to manage. However well supported and well informed he may be, the diabetic child will often find the mechanics of managing the disease irritating, the restriction it imposes irksome and the fact that he has a chronic disease distressing. This will often be reflected in his school work and his social life. He is likely to want to protest his ill luck and to draw attention to it, and he will certainly have discovered that this can be done effectively by failure to comply in any one of many ways up to and including leaving home without insulin or syringes!

Covert non-compliance, for example, the fudged urine tests, presents problems of detection as well as of management. All who encounter childhood diabetics soon learn the lesson, however, that most apparent aberrations in the disease can be accounted for simply if all details of management are carefully checked and double-checked.

Failures of Comprehension

These are often more the result of doctor failure than patient failure and, with some justice, the inadequately instructed patient returns to haunt his doctor. But even with the best will in the world it is impossible to prevent all errors. Among the more frequent are:

1. Failure to understand the effect of illness, emotional stress and other influences that disturb the diabetic equilibrium.

2. Failure to understand the duration of action of the insulin preparations used and the appropriate responses to poor control.

3. Confusion between marks on the insulin syringe (20 marks/ml) and units of insulin, or between 40 U/ml and 80 U/ml insulin preparations. (These recurring and unnecessary problems should be eradicated when the UK follows the USA and other countries in adopting a single insulin strength of 100 U/ml and suitable syringes.)

4. Problems with the insulin injections, especially the overuse of favoured areas from which absorption may be poor.

5. Problems with urine testing. It is particularly common with Clinitest to mistake the dirty green colour which follows a brief orange flush when heavy glycosuria is present as indicating 1 per cent (or 2 per cent with the 2-drop method) when in fact it indicates more than 2 per cent (or more than 5 per cent).

6. Misinterpretation of fluctuations in glycosuria as indicating inadequate rather than excessive insulin action. This is the swinging or Somogyi effect and, although clearly described by Somogyi in 1959, it is still ill understood and the cause of poor control in many diabetics. The child receiving an excessive dose of insulin shows hypoglycaemia (which may be brief and asymptomatic, especially at night) alternating with swings of blood sugar to high levels, often with some ketosis, as all the physiological mechanisms that raise blood sugar respond to the hypoglycaemia. The danger lies in the fact that the glycosuria and ketosis is thought by the diabetic to indicate the need for more insulin, thus initiating a vicious circle.

Illness

The diabetic child, especially if poorly controlled, is prone to develop intercurrent infections. Illness, especially febrile illness, causes catabolism and an increase in insulin requirement. Sensible parents can be taught to give small supplementary doses of soluble insulin as necessary.

Problems arise especially in the child who is vomiting. *To instruct such a child to stop his insulin may be lethal.* This fact is well known and yet two patients under our care have died in ketoacidosis at home after their doctors instructed them to stop their insulin until they were able to start eating again. The simplest approach is to give the routine dose of insulin and the usual dietary carbohydrate content, if necessary as sugar or glucose-containing fluids (dilute Coca Cola is usually acceptable: from the bottle it contains 30 g carbohydrate/100 ml), ignoring the fact that some may be vomited. If the urine tests show heavy glycosuria and especially if there is ketosis, supplementary doses of soluble insulin are necessary. In the unlikely event that there is no glycosuria, or even hypoglycaemia, a reduction in insulin dose is appropriate, but admission to hospital where an intravenous infusion of glucose can be given is probably wise.

Hypoglycaemia

Both the parents and the child should learn as soon as possible to recognize the individual but constant sequence of symptoms and signs that indicate hypoglycaemia. If the early warning symptoms, which are a consequence of catecholamine secretion, are detected, prompt feeding with quickly absorbed carbohydrate will prevent the onset of neuroglycopenic symptoms, which often include confusion and lack of co-operation.

In a few diabetic children hypoglycaemia may occur rapidly with little warning. Their parents should be supplied with glucagon ampoules and instructed to give 1 mg by intramuscular injection if the child refuses to accept or cannot swallow sugar by mouth. In addition, the diabetic regime should be carefully adjusted to avoid hypoglycaemia.

Occasional hypoglycaemia is inevitable if close diabetic control is attempted in all diabetic children, so every general practitioner should be willing to make occasional emergency visits to give intravenous glucose (0.5 to 1.0 g/kg).

Long-term Complications

The major long-term complications of diabetes have a vascular basis, either microvascular, including retinopathy and nephropathy, or macrovascular, in accelerated atherogenesis. As their development is closely related to the duration of diabetes they are seldom seen in childhood and will not be discussed. However, there is no longer any doubt that the development of these problems is delayed by good control, and it is largely for this reason that striving to improve control of childhood diabetes is so worthwhile.

Future Developments

Major developments in the management of diabetes seem imminent. In treatment these include the use of human insulin, produced by biosynthesis or chemical synthesis, oral delivery with liposomes or parenteral delivery closely mimicking physiological secretion, and transplantation of islets or whole pancreas.

Prevention of the disease may also prove feasible with identification of an at-risk population, protection against triggering pathogens and manipulation of the immune response. It certainly now seems reasonable, in talking to diabetic children and their parents, to express the hope that they will live in good health to see this disease finally conquered.

References

Farquhar, J. W., *Arch. Dis. Childh.*, 1979, **54**, 569.
Somogyi, M., *Am. J. Med.*, 1959, **26**, 169.

Further Reading

Craig, O., *Childhood Diabetes and its Management*, Butterworth, London, 1977.

15. ABC of Acute Problems

THIS chapter consists of a fragmented collection of short and necessarily dogmatic directions on the management of those acute emergencies in children which are most likely to be encountered by the general practitioner. We hope that these directions may prove useful for imaginary revision of the action appropriate in such crises and for support when synaptic transmission fails in the heat of the moment. You could keep a copy in your glove compartment, emergency bag, wallet or hat lining!

Dosage recommendations are, in most instances, expressed as mg/kg of bodyweight. In Table 15.1 approximate average weights at various ages through childhood are given. When a single dose is given, the usual adult dose is specified. Also shown in Table 15.1 are the approximate requirements for children expressed as a percentage of the adult dose. This method of dose calculation is generally reliable and safe.

Table 15.1. Average body weight and dose requirement in children.

Age	Approx. average weight kg	lb	Dose as percentage of adult dose
2 weeks	3	7	12
4 months	6	14	20
1 year	10	22	25
3 years	15	33	33
7 years	25	50	50
12 years	35	80	75

Anaphylaxis and Angio-oedema

Acute reactions may follow parenteral or oral exposure to a wide variety of allergens, notably drugs, foodstuffs, insect venoms and hyposensitization preparations.

First give 1 in 1,000 adrenaline, 0.2 to 0.5 ml subcutaneously, and massage to help absorption. Then give an antihistamine parenterally, such as chlorpheniramine (Piriton) 10 mg i.v. or i.m. If the symptoms do not immediately abate, arrange admission to hospital. If possible give oxygen and monitor the blood pressure. The administration of adrenaline can be repeated every 15 to 30 minutes if progressive airway obstruction or hypotension develop. A corticosteroid, such as hydrocortisone 200 mg i.v., can also be given; this will have no immediate effect but if symptoms prove to be prolonged, the sooner steroids are started the better. In hospital, tracheal intubation, infusion of plasma expanders with central venous pressure monitoring, and administration of adrenergic drugs may be required.

If the reaction is due to an injection or insect sting, a tourniquet can be applied to the affected limb and a similar dose of adrenaline injected subcutaneously at the site to slow absorption. The tourniquet must be removed 10 to 15 minutes later.

After recovery, remember that hyposensitization may be needed.

Asthma (see chapter 6)

When an asthmatic attack fails to respond to oral or inhaled betamimetic drugs, subcutaneous administration of terbutaline (Bricanyl) 10 μg per kg, or salbutamol (Ventolin) 8 μg per kg will often be successful. In more severe cases admission to hospital is necessary. In addition to unresponsiveness to sympathomimetic drugs, the following findings indicate that hospital admission is urgent:

1. Cyanosis, for which oxygen should be given as soon as possible.

2. Decreased respiratory effort due to exhaustion. This results in decreased air entry and a relatively quiet chest which can be mistaken for improvement.

3. Tachycardia greater than 180 beats per minute, hyper- or hypotension, pulsus paradoxus, shock.

4. Confusion or unconsciousness.

Therapy before transfer should include the following:

1. Bronchodilators. These should be administered as already described, but with care if betamimetic or theophylline compounds have already been given, and in the presence of cyanosis or cardiovascular collapse.

2. Oxygen. Children can safely be given oxygen because their respiratory drive is always CO_2 sensitive. Children with status asthmaticus are always hypoxic and their anxiety as well as their asthma may improve when oxygen is given. Ensure that the ambulance also carries oxygen.

3. Corticosteroids. Even by intravenous injection in large doses, steroids take at least an hour to have an effect on bronchospasm and four to six hours before major benefit is achieved. Nevertheless, give hydrocortisone 200 mg i.v. to all severe asthmatics as soon as possible because the effect will probably have started by the time the patient reaches hospital and the action of bronchodilator drugs is potentiated in the presence of high circulating levels of cortisol.

Figure 15.1. *The two-handed method of cardiac massage. Note that both hands encircle the chest and both thumbs are used for cardiac compression.*

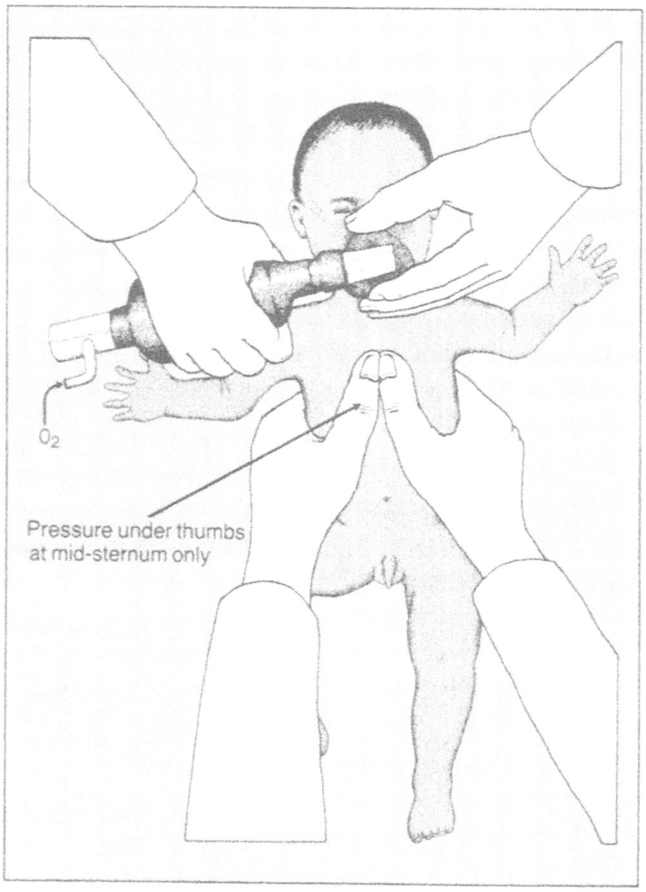

On no account should sedatives of any sort be given to children with severe asthma however distressed they may be.

Ataxia

Acute ataxia in children is most frequently due to ingestion of drugs or alcohol. Check the drug history of all family members and also check the drinks' cupboard. Keep in mind the odder forms of intoxication, such as solvent sniffing. The drugs most frequently involved are the anticonvulsants, sedatives and piperazine, which is notorious for the induction of 'worm wobble'.

Other causes of ataxia include encephalitis, especially that following chickenpox, and space-occupying lesions in the posterior fossa.

Burns

First cool the affected area, ideally by immersion in water, especially if it is a chemical burn, or by the repeated application of cold water compresses. Hospital admission will be required for all but the smallest full thickness burns, for all those involving the face, hands or perineum, and for burns of any type involving more than 10 per cent of the body surface. If the burn was due to a fire, smoke inhalation and burning of the respiratory tract may be a major problem. Such children will require oxygen on their way to hospital.

Cardiac and Respiratory Arrest

If confronted with an apparently dead child it is always worth attempting cardiopulmonary resuscitation if there is the slightest chance that this may prove successful. This is particularly true of drowning in cold water (see next page) in which neurologically intact survival has been reported after as long as 40 minutes submersion.

Respiratory Arrest

The first action is to clear the airway. Having ascertained that no obstruction is present, the jaw should be held forward and the neck extended. If there is no spontaneous respiratory movement, mouth to mouth ventilation can then be given, with the lips covering both the mouth and nose in infants and small children. Excessive inflation pressure must be avoided because this can cause pneumothorax. More satisfactory ventilation can, of course, be achieved with an oral airway and a ventilatory bag if these are available (Figure 15.1). Laryngoscopy and tracheal intubation should be attempted only by those who are skilled in the technique because clumsy attempts may damage the airway and add to the respiratory problems. However ventilation is given, it is essential to ensure that the chest is moving due to inflation of the lungs and not simply due to inflation of the stomach. Oxygen-enriched air should be used if possible.

Cardiac Arrest

If the pulse is absent or inadequate, external cardiac massage should be started simultaneously with assisted ventilation. Four beats of cardiac massage are given for each lung inflation. In small babies the thorax should be encircled by the hands, allowing the thumbs to depress the sternum against the resistance of the fingers (Figure 15.1). Prodding the sternum with two fingers does not produce an adequate impulse. In older children sufficient force must be applied to the sternum to give a good femoral pulse. Fortunately in children the rib cage is extremely compliant so it is difficult to fracture ribs or damage intrathoracic or intra-abdominal viscera. If available, sodium bicarbonate 5 to 10 mmol/kg should be given intravenously (8.4 per cent sodium bicarbonate contains 1 mmol/ml), and an intracardiac injection of adrenaline, 0.5 to 1 ml of 1 in 1,000, should also be given before resuscitation is abandoned.

If no heart beat is achieved within 10 minutes and more sophisticated resuscitation facilities are not available, further attempts will be of no avail except in hypothermic children.

Coma

The causes of coma in children are listed in Table 15.2, with the incidence of these conditions seen in a Canadian paediatric neurology service over a 15-month period from September 1974 (Seshia et al. 1977). It is often possible to establish the diagnosis clinically; if no explanation is apparent postictal coma and drug ingestion are most likely. The blood glucose should always be checked in cases of unexplained unconsciousness and Dextrostix testing strips are a most useful portable diagnostic aid for the general practitioner. Remember that alcohol ingestion sometimes causes profound hypoglycaemia in children and that, even if the members of the household know of no drugs to which the child had access, visiting elderly relatives often carry with them a portable pharmacopoeia.

In comatose patients it is first essential to ensure the patency of the airway, the adequacy of ventilation and the integrity of the circulation. Having ascertained that respiratory and cardiac function are adequate, the child should be placed in the coma position, semiprone and with the head slightly down, to maintain cerebral perfusion and prevent inhalation of secretions.

Table 15.2. Causes of coma in childhood. (Drug ingestion, head injury and neurosurgical problems, such as extradural haemorrhage and tumour are excluded).

Cause	No. of cases in series
Intracranial infection (meningitis/encephalitis)	26
Anoxia, ischaemia (post-cardiac arrest)	18
Postictal	11
Metabolic (hypoglycaemia, severe dehydration, Addisonian, liver failure, diabetes	11
Severe septicaemia	3
Intracranial vascular lesion	3

Cough

Persistent unremitting cough is most frequently due to an inhaled foreign body but consider also pertussis, asthma, inhaled irritants and pulmonary oedema.

Croup

See respiratory obstruction, page 108.

Dehydration

The assessment of dehydration is described in chapter 11. All children, especially infants, with serious dehydration (5 per cent or greater) require admission to hospital. Intravenous rehydration will be necessary and the only useful treatment which can be started before admission is administration of oxygen to minimize the effects of hypoxia secondary to low cardiac output.

Diabetes (see chapter 14)

Severe diabetic ketoacidosis leads to precoma and coma and such children require urgent admission to hospital. No specific therapy should be given in the home. If the child is unconscious, the first aid measures already described for coma should be instituted. In early diabetic ketoacidosis the child urgently requires fluid and insulin. We have seen more than one death directly resulting from instructions to stop the insulin in diabetic children with persistent vomiting.

Drowning

Even children who are conscious when fished from the water should be assessed in hospital because the inhalation of fresh or salt water may cause secondary pulmonary problems.

The airway should be cleared of particulate matter

and oxygen administered. If respiratory or cardiac arrest has taken place, resuscitation should be attempted. It is worth checking the pupillary reflexes, since some apparently dead victims of drowning are in fact alive and retain their pupillary reactions despite profound vagally induced bradycardia and hypotension.

Resuscitation must be continued until admission to hospital. Intact survival has been reported after prolonged cardiopulmonary resuscitation, especially in patients who were immersed in very cold water (Siebke et al. 1975).

Dystonia

Dystonic movements of various types, including oculogyric crises, are increasingly seen in children given phenothiazines (e.g. Stemetil, Fentazin) or other drugs (e.g. Maxolon) as antiemetics or sedatives. Such a reaction should be suspected in any child who presents with a history of an acute movement disorder particularly if the head and eyes are affected. It is often at first suspected that the child has hysterical symptoms or epilepsy. The abnormal movements respond rapidly to an antiparkinsonian agent, e.g. benztropine (Cogentin) 0.5 to 1 mg i.v. The dose can be repeated if necessary.

Electrocution

Before approaching the patient, especially if there is water around, as in a bathroom, switch off the power. The management is essentially that of cardiorespiratory arrest and burns, but remember that a pulseless patient may have ventricular fibrillation and may revert to sinus rhythm with a sharp blow to the praecordium.

Epistaxis (see Haemorrhage)

Fits (see chapter 8)

It is prudent to admit all children to hospital after a first fit, including a febrile fit, unless the attending doctor is absolutely confident that there is no underlying intracranial infection, metabolic abnormality or space-occupying lesion. The clinical signs of meningitis are unreliable in infants under two years of age, especially in the postictal state. If such an infant is to be managed at home a further visit within a few hours to confirm the absence of meningitis is mandatory. Hypoglycaemia must be excluded, especially if the fit occurred in the fasting state or there were associated signs of catecholamine excess. A Dextrostix test should be performed on all children who have had a first or non-febrile fit and on those children prone to hypoglycaemia, such as diabetics. The fundi should be carefully examined in any child who has had a fit, an examination which is often difficult to achieve even under ideal circumstances.

Fortunately children rarely injure themselves in fits but clearly they must be removed from situations of danger. The airway must be maintained but spoons, wedges, pieces of wood and especially fingers should not be inserted between the teeth because the tongue is usually bitten in the first spasm and teeth (and fingertips) are more likely to be lost than preserved by intervention. The child should be placed in the coma position and oxygen given if available.

The fit should be stopped as soon as possible. Give diazepam (Valium) by slow intravenous injection until the fit ceases or an initial dose of 0.25 mg/kg has been given. In the circumstances this can, of course, be difficult to administer and, although intramuscular Valium is too slow-acting, it has recently been shown that rectal instillation of the parenteral solution is rapidly effective. An injection of 1 ml (5 mg) should be given into the rectum with a small syringe, and the buttocks squeezed to avoid leakage. An alternative treatment is paraldehyde which is given by deep intramuscular injection in a dosage of 1 ml per year of age to a maximum of 10 ml. It is not necessary to use a glass syringe if the drug is given as soon as it is drawn up.

If the fit is not controlled within 15 minutes, the anticonvulsant can be repeated. Close observation must be maintained even after the fit has ceased because the anticonvulsant may cause respiratory depression.

A prolonged fit is an urgent indication for hospital admission.

Haemorrhage

Major haemorrhage from any site is an indication for hospital admission. Bleeding should be controlled by firm local pressure with a dressing, which may need to be held in place by hand. Tourniquets should not be used to control bleeding from limbs since they are likely merely to substitute ischaemic limb loss for haemorrhagic hypotension.

Nose bleeding can usually be controlled in the home by sitting the child upright, instructing him to breathe through his mouth and applying firm pressure with a cold pack to the nostrils continuously for five minutes by the clock.

In a child with unexplained bleeding of an unusually severe degree an underlying disorder, such as a bleeding diathesis or hypertension, should be considered.

Head Injury

Children are constantly falling over and banging their heads. If they do not lose consciousness and have no subsequent symptoms other than local pain, no medical evaluation is needed, or indeed sought, in most instances. A more difficult problem is presented by the child who is briefly concussed or develops symptoms, such as marked pallor, lethargy or vomiting, shortly after the injury. Such children should be carefully examined, including the fundi. If no abnormality is found, it seems reasonable for them to be observed at home. The parents can be instructed to wake them once or twice in the night to check that they are normally rousable. If the circumstances and severity of the head injury were uncertain, if the child was unconscious for more than a matter of seconds, if any neurological abnormality is present or if the symptoms are unduly prolonged, referral to hospital for skull x-ray, full neurological examination and probable admission for observation is mandatory. Remember the fact, only too well known to all neurosurgeons, that the most frequent, preventable and remediable cause of deterioration after head injury is airway obstruction.

Hiccough

If the usual tricks of eating a teaspoonful of sugar, drinking from the wrong side of a cup or scaring the wits out of the child do not work, consider intrathoracic or intra-abdominal conditions which may cause diaphragmatic irritation. Chlorpromazine 1 mg/kg i.v. may relieve intractable hiccough.

Hyperpyrexia

The higher a child's temperature above 40°C (104°F), the greater the danger of fits and brain damage. The temperature should therefore be controlled as soon as possible. The cause must be sought and treated and hydration sustained by an adequate fluid intake, allowing for increased insensible loss. The temperature should be lowered by giving aspirin, orally or rectally, 10 mg/kg every 4 to 6 hours or paracetamol orally 5 mg/kg every 4 to 6 hours. The naked child should be tepid sponged using warm water at a temperature of 75° to 80°F. Colder water causes peripheral vasconstriction and shivering and may thereby increase the temperature. If there is vascular collapse from dehydration cooling by tepid sponging will be ineffective until the plasma volume is expanded and peripheral perfusion increased.

Any child with a temperature above 40.5°C should be admitted to hospital. Serious bacterial infections, such as septicaemia, meningitis and pneumonia, are common with this degree of fever and, in addition, the severely hyperpyrexic child may need cooling by the controlled use of alpha-blocking drugs combined with intravenous fluid therapy. Remember that severe degrees of hyperpyrexia can occur in healthy infants who have been dressed up for the cold and then left near a radiator or stove or in direct sunlight through the window of a closed room or car.

Hyperventilation

In a child who is overbreathing, consider metabolic acidosis (due to diabetic ketoacidosis, gastroenteritis, renal failure or other metabolic problems) asthma or parenchymal pulmonary disease, aspirin overdose, intracranial problems and hysterical hyperventilation. The organic problems clearly require urgent investigation and treatment. The symptoms of hysterical hyperventilation are due to respiratory alkalaemia and this can be reversed by breathing a 5 per cent carbon-dioxide/95 per cent oxygen mixture or, more simply, by rebreathing from a paper bag or balloon in such a way that dissipation of the accumulating carbon dioxide is prevented.

Hypoglycaemia (see chapter 14)

The use of Dextrostix testing strips has been mentioned previously and all general practitioners should carry them to help in the evaluation of potentially hypoglycaemic symptoms including strange behaviour, fits and coma. If there is any doubt about the reading obtained because, for instance, the testing strips may have deteriorated, it is always worthwhile to obtain a simultaneous 'control' value by pricking oneself or the nearest apparently normoglycaemic victim! In symptomatic hypoglycaemia the blood glucose will be less than 45 mg per 100 ml (2.5 mmol/l). If the child is conscious and can swallow, give 10 to 20 g of glucose or household sugar (two to four heaped teaspoons or sugar lumps) in a little water. If there is no improvement within 5 to 10 minutes, repeat the dose. If the child is unable or unwilling to swallow, give 50 per cent dextrose 0.5 to 1 ml/kg intravenously. Except in conditions where hepatic glycogen is not available, parenteral glucagon rapidly raises the blood glucose; give 1 mg (1 ampoule) by intravenous or intramuscular injection. The parents of diabetic children prone to hypoglycaemia should be instructed in the use of glucagon.

Encourage the child who has recovered from hypoglycaemia to have a meal and arrange observation if recurrence seems likely.

Hypothermia

Children with a core body temperature of 35°C or less require hospital admission both for controlled rewarming and, in those in whom hypothermia is not simply due to exposure, for exclusion of underlying pathology, such as sepsis or hypothyroidism. Until admission can be arranged, wrap the child in warmed clothing and blankets to insulate as fully as possible. A silver swaddler is extremely effective if available. Keep the child in as warm surroundings as possible but do not apply direct heat from hot water bottles, electric blankets, etc., because these may burn the poorly perfused skin of a hypothermic patient. Immersion in warm water should probably be avoided because it may cause an initial fall in core temperature with ill effects on cardiac function as cold blood from the surface begins to recirculate. Keep the child lying horizontal to minimize the effects of hypotension and remember the strong association, especially in infants, between hypothermia and hypoglycaemia.

Table 15.3. Telephone numbers of Poison Control Centres.

Belfast	0232-40503
Cardiff	0222-492233
Dublin	0001-45588
Edinburgh	031-229 2477
Leeds	0532-32799
London	01-407 7600
Manchester	061-740 2254
Newcastle-upon-Tyne	0632-25131

Inhalation of Foreign Body

An object in the back of the throat can often be removed with fingers or a pair of forceps. If this fails and the child is showing signs of airway obstruction, the object may be removed by upending the child and pounding on his back or, alternatively, suddenly compressing the upper abdomen to force the diaphragm upward and blast the object out of the airway (Heimlich manoeuvre). If all else fails and there is severe obstruction, consider the measures listed under 'Respiratory Obstruction' below.

After such an episode the child should be x-rayed and, if necessary, observed in hospital in case pieces of the foreign body are retained or complications, such as oedema of the airway and aspiration pneumonia, occur.

Poisoning

The main measure required to cut the distressing toll of childhood poisoning is, of course, prevention.

All general practitioners should be armed with a copy of Matthew and Lawson's useful little book, *The Treatment of Common Acute Poisonings* (1975), and should know the telephone number of the local Poison Control Centre (Table 15.3) where comprehensive advice can be obtained day and night. Drug and toxin ingestion should always be considered in the differential diagnosis of odd central nervous system symptoms and coma.

The first essential is to obtain as accurate a history as possible of what and how much was ingested. If it is absolutely certain that only a small amount of a relatively harmless drug or other substance has been taken, a well child can be observed at home. If larger quantities or mixtures of noxious substances may have been taken, if there is drowsiness or any other symptom, and if any quantity of notorious substances, such as iron, aspirin, paracetamol, barbiturates, antidepressants, all corrosive household and petroleum products or paraquat is involved, then admission to hospital for treatment and observation is essential.

Only the following measures are recommended in the home. First remove the child from the source of poison or vice versa. Retain a specimen for identification or chemical analysis. Second, wash all poison off the skin, especially if a corrosive or petroleum product has been taken. Third, induce vomiting in children who are fully conscious and who have taken in the previous two hours (four hours in the case of aspirin) drugs or poisons other than corrosives and petroleum products. Vomiting is best induced by putting the child over an adult's knee in a 'spanking' position and irritating the throat with a blunt-ended wooden spoon or other suitable implement. A little warm water or milk will give the child something to vomit. Keep the vomit for analysis. Chemical emetic agents are less desirable because they are slower, may not work and produce toxic side-effects. The best is ipecac syrup, 15 ml for the child over one year, followed by some water. If vomiting is delayed, it can usually be induced by joggling the child up and down a few times. Some parents still try to induce vomiting with strong salt solutions which are particularly dangerous.

If the child is semiconscious or unconscious, aspiration is a real danger and no attempt should be made to induce vomiting. The child should be managed as described for coma.

Respiratory Obstruction

Two causes of acute respiratory obstruction have been discussed earlier in this chapter under Anaphylaxis and Inhalation of Foreign Body. In children, the commonest cause of upper respiratory tract obstruction is infective croup, which, in about 95 per cent of cases is due to viral laryngotracheitis and in 5 per cent to *Haemophilus* epiglottitis. These conditions are discussed in chapter 4. Complete airway obstruction is rare in viral croup but common in epiglottitis, which is characterized by the older age-group affected, the more acute and prostrating illness, the dysphagia and drooling, and the muffled rather than hoarse voice. Suspected cases of epiglottitis should be transferred immediately to a hospital with full emergency facilities. No attempt should be made to examine the upper airway because this may provoke complete obstruction. The only worthwhile emergency procedure is to pocket a wide-bore cannula, to put the child in the nearest car with an assistant to help him maintain the sitting position he will prefer and to give him oxygen if available, and to convey him as quickly as possible to the nearest suitable unit. Viral croup, in contrast, is a less acute problem which can often be managed at home. The airway obstruction is much more slowly progressive and usually self-limiting. If there is progressive respiratory difficulty as shown by restlessness, feeding difficulty, increased respiratory effort and increasing tachypnoea and tachycardia, admission to hospital will, of course, be necessary.

If total obstruction of the airway occurs and cannot be relieved by less drastic measures, an emergency airway can be established by inserting a wide-bore Medicut (12 to 16 french gauge) or similar cannula through the cricothyroid membrane as illustrated in Figure 15.2. This technique will provide an airway adequate to sustain life during a journey to hospital where emergency intubation or tracheotomy can be performed.

Figure 15.2. *Site for insertion of Medicut when managing acute upper airway obstruction (from Clarke and Cochrane 1975, with permission).*

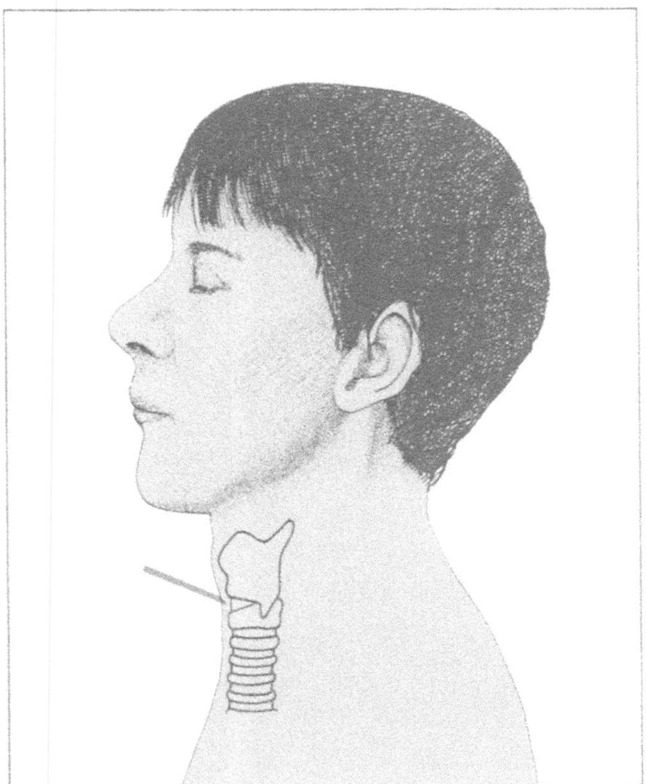

Septicaemia

The meningococcus is the commonest cause of septicaemia in children and a clue to the diagnosis is usually provided by the presence of skin haemorrhages, at first tiny petechiae (see chapter 13, figure 13.1) some of which may later develop into extensive ecchymotic lesions (Figure 15.3). Pneumococcal septicaemia may also present as an acute fulminant illness especially in children who have had a splenectomy. Gram-negative septicaemia tends to occur in children with underlying renal or alimentary tract problems or an immunodeficiency state, congenital or acquired.

All children in whom septicaemia is suspected must be admitted to hospital immediately, before antibiotic therapy is commenced. If the child is hypotensive (systolic blood pressure of less than 80 mm Hg) hydrocortisone 200 mg i.v. or i.m. should be given. During transit, oxygen should be given if peripheral vasoconstriction has occurred.

Stings or Snakebite

Insect stings in Britain rarely pose a problem other than local discomfort. Anaphylactic reactions are fortunately rare and have been considered previously in this chapter. Bee stings are alkaline and wasp, hornet and ant stings are acidic. Application of a dilute solution of an appropriate acid, such as vinegar, or alkali, such as baking soda, may therefore be soothing. A local antihistamine cream may also help.

The viper is the only snake in the UK with a poisonous bite. The dramatic lancing, sucking, spitting and tourniquets beloved of Hollywood producers are positively harmful. Cleanse the wound, immobilize the limb and give tetanus toxoid. Children with systemic symptoms should be referred to hospital for management.

Figure 15.3. *The haemorrhagic rash of established meningococcal septicaemia.*

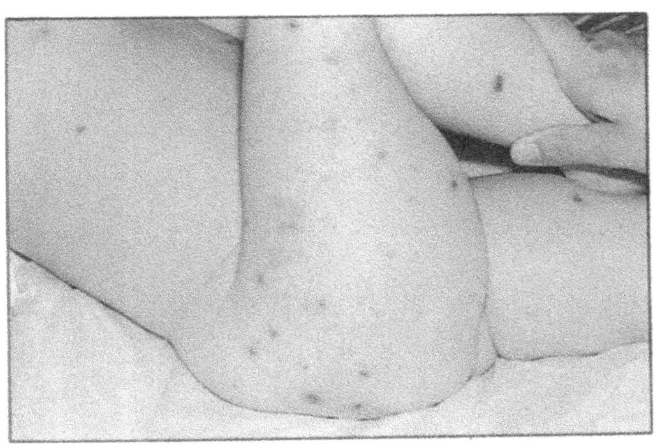

Screaming

An infant who screams inconsolably for hours is likely to be in pain. Most mothers soon learn to differentiate their infant's cry of pain from that of anger. Teething seldom seems to be sufficiently painful to cause real misery. Possible serious diagnoses include unsuspected fractures (remember nonaccidental injury), acute otitis media, acute arthritis or osteomyelitis, intussusception, incarcerated hernia and raised intracranial pressure from any cause. Careful examination will usually reveal the problem but sometimes hospital assessment will be required for diagnosis or simply for the relief of anxiety. Sedation of the really inconsolable child at home before a diagnosis is established may result in serious disease being missed and, when the sedation wears off and the screaming starts again, may expose the child to maltreatment by his overwrought parents.

References

Clarke, S. W. and Cochrane, G. M., *Practitioner,* 1975, **215**, 340.

Matthew, H. and Lawson, A. A. H., *Treatment of the Common Acute Poisonings,* 3rd edition, Churchill Livingstone, Edinburgh, 1975.

Seshia, S. S., Seshia, M. M. K. and Sachdeva, R. K., *Dev. Med. Child Neurol.,* 1977, **19**, 614.

Siebke, H., Breiveik, H., Rød, T. and Lind, B., *Lancet,* 1975, **i**, 1275.

Further Reading

Black, J. A., *Paediatric Emergencies,* Butterworth, London, 1979.

Symposium on pediatric emergencies, *Pediatr. Clin. North Am.,* 1979, **26**.

16. Behaviour Problems

BEHAVIOUR problems in children are universal, indeed they are essential. Friction inevitably results from the infinitely complex process through which each child adjusts to his own emotional, intellectual and physical development while simultaneously forming and testing his relationships with his family, his peers and others. Indeed, it seems remarkable how smoothly most children mature and find their place in society and how seldom their early experiments in behaviour cause more than transient and acceptable aggravation.

Parents, teachers, doctors and all in contact with children inevitably gain experience of the minor problems which arise from this adjustment process. In general they also share a lack of formal instruction on the management of such problems and so establish their own methods by trial and error! The comments offered in this chapter are derived largely from just such empirical experience gained in our roles as general paediatricians and, perhaps more important, as fathers. They are not based on any unified concept of child development or any single school of thought on management and, indeed, if any professional child psychiatrist or psychologist should inadvertently stray onto these pages, we warn him that further reading may prove hazardous to his health!

Fortunately, since few general practitioners or paediatricians have either the time or the skill to undertake such work, the management of behaviour problems in children only seldom requires in-depth psychiatric assessment and prolonged psychotherapy. The cornerstone of management is simple explanation and reassurance, in the course of which it is often necessary to expound convincingly a few straightforward principles of child development and child-rearing. We will therefore summarize the facts we like to emphasize in this context and will then proceed to discuss briefly some specific problems and some principles of management, indicating when it seems to us desirable to enlist more expert help. A good general account of behaviour problems is given in Illingworth's excellent book, *The Normal Child* (1975).

The Evolution of Behaviour

The development of behaviour through childhood can be considered in four stages.

Infancy, from Birth to 1 Year

The infant is dependent on his mother or a mother-substitute for all his needs. At first he is provided only with a signal for distress but he soon learns to demonstrate pleasure with smiles, coos and movements. This is the oral stage of the classical psychoanalytic model of development and his main satisfaction is feeding. The unique importance of attachment to his mother from the first minute of life is increasingly recognized and, as the months pass, he is wont to express forcibly his resentment when separated from this central figure in his life. Problematic behaviour is virtually synonymous with excessive crying and generally results from either feeding or sleeping difficulties.

Preschool, 1 to 5 Years

The child's increasing awareness and newly acquired mobility permit him to explore the world of which he is the centre and to taste the exciting possibilities of independence. The acquisition of speech infinitely extends the range of his social contacts. He learns to co-operate with others but also becomes aware that his wishes may conflict with theirs. He is determined to do things his way and a struggle for dominance with his parents occurs as he repeatedly tests his power to manipulate his environment. Unopposed, he may soon run the household absolutely. Around this primary confrontation with his parents intricate subplots may develop with the intrusion of siblings (especially those newly arrived) and others: the child first experiences jealousy and rivalry; he becomes aware of his sexual role and sexual curiosity and erotic feelings arise; he begins to develop a conscience and a sense of guilt. Behaviour disturbance continues to centre on problems of feeding and sleeping to which are added difficulties in toilet training, temper tantrums, separation anxiety and other fears, rational and irrational.

Primary School, 5 to 11 Years

During these years the child directs his main energies to the process of coming to terms with the wider world outside the family. He explores relationships with his peers and finds where he fits into his expanded concept of the universe. Formal learning occupies him more and more and he is continually testing his intellect and personality against those of his peers. This is the stage of latency in which erotic feelings and conflicts are thought to subside before reappearing in adolescence. Behaviour problems centre around the difficulties of fitting into a group and mastering the difficult basic educational skills.

Secondary School, 11 to 16 Years

The child's world once again changes comprehensively in this stage of adolescence. He must come to terms with the adult world while coping with the greater demands placed on him and the internal upheavals that accompany puberty, a condition memorably described by Philip Roth in *Portnoy's Complaint* as 'a disorder in which strongly held ethical and altruistic impulses are perpetually warring with extreme sexual longings'! During this time the adolescent must start the process of separating from his parents, taking with him some and rejecting other parts of the emotional and behavioural baggage he has acquired during his childhood; he must prepare himself for a job or for further education and he must come to terms with his sexual identity. It is hardly surprising that these years are so difficult and fraught with possibilities of disaster. Behaviour problems are generally expressed in rebelliousness, rejection of the standards and goals set by parents and teachers, sexual difficulties and delinquency.

The Principles of Child Rearing

For the purposes of discussion with parents the essentials of child rearing can be reduced to four simple principles.

Children Need Love

Children are emotionally clear-sighted in matters concerning themselves and are able to sense real from phoney affection, from whatever quarter each may come. As dogs and horses are reputed to do (we have previously mentioned the analogies of paediatrics with veterinary matters), they detect dislike, fear, uncertainty and distrust and respond negatively to them. Behaviour disturbance does not thrive on a diet of love and acceptance. At one level parental love should be unconditional but the natural fluctuations of affectionate feeling at a more superficial level can usefully be expressed. Indeed, to conceal these responses is wrong and will deprive the child of the vital knowledge of the effect his behaviour has on others. Equally, parents must be allowed to feel without guilt the extreme exasperation that the parental state so often engenders. Many find great relief in the reassurance that an occasional feeling of aggression towards their children is entirely normal.

Children do not Listen, They Copy

Children model their behaviour on that they see around them and, just as they ignore words if they contradict actions, they ignore actions if they contradict motives. Their intellectual comprehension of adult motives is, of course, limited but the accuracy of their instinctive appreciation of interactions between people is disconcertingly acute. Conversely, although the motives of children are usually apparent if a little empathy is used, many parents fail to make such simple interpretation and are, for instance, greatly surprised to be told that their 'naughty' child is simply trying to draw attention to himself because of an underlying sense of insecurity.

It is the child's need to copy which make a stable parent figure of each sex and a loving relationship between these two adults such important factors in development. When two such figures in such a relationship cannot be provided as a model for the child, the stable love of one parent is a good second best. The strong tendency of children to repeat the patterns of their parents, from broken marriages through suicide to child abuse, seems likely to be determined far more by environment than by heredity.

Encouragement is Better than Punishment

Changes in behaviour are far more likely to be achieved by positive reward than by negative punishment. It is common experience that punishment of a child can escalate to disturbing levels of physical or mental cruelty without achieving the desired behaviour from the victim. Love and attention are the rewards children of all ages appreciate most. There is no doubt, however, that these can sometimes be reinforced effectively with bribery of a more tangible nature! This is, of course, the basis of behaviour therapy.

Rules are Necessary

Children of all ages need absolute limits set on their freedom and made clear without equivocation. For younger children these limits may be determined largely by personal safety ('you must not play on the railway line') and for adolescents by the law of the land ('you must go to school'). Within these outer limits are large areas for negotiation where consistency, rationality and a measure of give and take (including a willingness on the parental side to make strategic retreats when out-manoeuvred!) are necessary. Concern for the child himself should be the evident principle underlying most rules. Older children also require an ethical code; they need to know the rules of moral behaviour that their parents would wish them to set. Here parents may expose a credibility gap between wish and performance in their own behaviour, which children pick up with unerring instinct. With luck, by this age they may have begun to appreciate how difficult it is to realize higher aspirations, and their inevitable (and necessary) disillusion with their parents may be leavened with some sympathy and understanding. If an over-riding principle of kindness and consideration for others has emerged from all the child has been taught, he may remember to include his parents in the beneficiaries. (Is that ribald laughter we hear from readers who are the parents of teenagers?! Ah well, there's no harm in hoping!)

Specific Behaviour Problems

Feeding Problems

Failure to Eat

Feeding is the activity that most frequently brings parent and child into painful conflict. The complaint is usually some variation of the theme that the child 'never eats'. The subject of this complaint is almost invariably well-nourished and sometimes obese! All children discover at some time the pleasing fact that refusal to eat elicits a strong reaction from their parents. Persistent refusal often leads, in a classic description by Joseph Brennemann, to 'coaxing, teasing, urging, cajoling, spoofing, wheedling, begging, shaming, scolding, nagging, threatening, bribing, punishing, pointing out and demonstrating the excellence of the food, weeping or pretending to weep, playing the fool, singing a song, telling a story or showing a picture book, turning on the radio, beating a drum, even having the grandmother dance a jig'! The pleasure to be gained from these delightful parental contortions is, however, strongly counterbalanced by the resulting sense of hunger. Except in the adolescent with anorexia nervosa, the need to eat invariably prevails. All the parents need to achieve is convincingly feigned indifference. Unfortunately, for reasons of their own, they often find this difficult or impossible; they may be genuinely anxious that the child will be harmed by undernutrition, they may have totally unrealistic ideas about the amount of food the child needs or they may harbour at a more or less conscious level ambivalent feelings about the child. These problems often need to be explored before they can take the simple action necessary to start to return the child's feeding habits to an acceptable pattern.

Obesity

In contrast to the problem of failure to eat, obesity is generally presented to the doctor as an organic rather than a behavioural disorder. This is probably appropriate as increasing evidence indicates that many overweight children consume no more calories than their slim peers. The problem thus lies more with their genetic metabolic endowment than with culpable greed. Sufficient calorie restriction results in weight loss in all obese people. However, such stringency is occasionally necessary that it proves virtually impossible for even the minority of children, who are well-motivated, to lose weight. In some families with obese children, however, enormous meals are regularly consumed and moderate dietary restriction may result in a gratifying loss of weight.

Sleeping Problems

These are also extremely common through childhood and generally present with the simple complaint 'he won't sleep'. This can introduce a variety of problems, such as a baby who cries persistently at night, a toddler with night terrors, a schoolchild who refuses to go to bed or persistently wakes, or an adolescent with sleep-walking. Clearly many factors may play a part in causing these problems including the child's intrinsic need for sleep (often far less than the parents suppose), the ease with which he wakes, the bedtime routine and sleeping environment, the child's anxieties and those of his parents. Sleep disturbance often follows obviously disrupting experiences, such as admission to hospital.

Children differ remarkably in their need for sleep and, except with hypnotic drugs which have only a limited place in management (see page 116), it is no more possible to force a child to sleep than to feed. A sensible objective is to persuade the child to spend a reasonable number of hours in bed each night either asleep or, if awake, entertaining himself quietly. This desirable end is generally achieved by ensuring the child is ready for sleep at his bedtime, that he knows and accepts (and preferably enjoys) the bedtime routine and that he is not afraid of nameless night terrors or other spectres. The management of sleep disturbance in the young child has recently been well reviewed by Bax (1980).

Problems of Excretion

In the absence of negative forces and in the presence of

mild positive encouragement children will become dry and clean as soon as their neuromuscular control permits. Having acquired these vital social skills, only rarely and under considerable provocation will they lose them. The most potent force likely to disrupt this natural process is excessive zeal on the part of parents for their child to achieve continence before he is neurologically ready to do so. This invests the whole matter, already of great and natural interest to the child at this stage of development, with far too much emotional charge whether applied to 'failure' or 'success'. As the child becomes aware of his excretory processes, he should learn that it is not a matter of the greatest importance and the sooner he is able to achieve continence and look after his own needs the better; meanwhile nappies are simply a necessary expedient. All children delight in becoming independent. The appropriate response to a child's first correctly placed offering should be a long way short of a family celebration in full evening dress with presentation of an inscribed pot!

Attempts to train children earlier than their neuromuscular control allows often lead to unnecessary problems. Although with persistence some degree of reflex sphincter control can be achieved in younger children by enthroning them at frequent intervals, it is unreasonable to expect a child to be out of nappies by day before two years and by night about six months later. Regularly sitting the child on the pot before this age is probably a harmless routine and can save a lot of washing as long as the mother realizes that such 'control' is merely reflex conditioning and does not become anxious if it is lost for some time before the control is again established. When the child begins to indicate his own needs he must, of course, be offered suitable facilities.

Persistent primary enuresis and encopresis in undisturbed children are likely to be due to organic causes, most frequently simple delay in the achievement of adequate sphincter control, often a familial characteristic. If the child does show psychological disturbance this may, of course, be the result rather than the cause of the problem. In addition, organic problems, such as urinary tract infection or constipation with overflow, must be excluded before wetting or soiling is ascribed to psychological disturbance. When these problems are psychologically determined, they are usually part of a much more widespread disturbance of behaviour and require full psychological investigation and appropriate therapy.

Temper Tantrums

Uncontrolled bouts of fury are not uncommon in normal children from about 18 months to 3 years and, in the context of otherwise normal behaviour, need not be a cause for great anxiety. Management should be along the usual lines of firm, consistent and dispassionate handling and, if the child fails to gain any rewards from this highly undesirable behaviour pattern, he will soon abandon it. If tantrums continue to occur they are of more worrying import, especially if they are a feature of a more general behaviour disturbance.

Masturbation

Most children engage in some self-stimulation around 2 to 6 years of age. They tend to do so when alone, presumably for lack of a more entertaining pastime rather than from any inappropriate sense of shame. Many parents need reassuring that such behaviour is normal and self-limiting. Some still fear that masturbation in the adolescent child may prove physically and morally harmful. Such ideas die hard and it was only 120 years ago that Dr Henry Maudsley, one of the more enlightened psychiatrists of the 19th century, concluded a lecture to the Harveian Society on the subject of masturbation in adolescent boys by stating that treatment was hopeless for this 'serious mental disease, the sooner the victim sinks to his degraded rest the better for himself and the better for the world which is well rid of him'.

Habits

At some time most children develop repetitive habits, such as thumb-sucking or finger-nail biting, which worry or distress their parents. The great majority are harmless and transient. Since most such habits are probably devices to relieve mild anxiety, a guiding principle in management is to avoid increasing anxiety by drawing too much attention to the problem. The most useful recommendation, therefore, is for the parents to grit their teeth and avoid badgering the child while awaiting spontaneous resolution of the habit. The same principles apply, although rather more parental self-control is needed, to children with tics and habit spasms. Repetitive rocking and head-banging are rather more worrying. They are particularly common in deprived and retarded children although they do occur in entirely normal children. Once again there is little specific treatment to offer apart from reassurance and advice on padding the cot, moving it away from the connecting wall with the neighbours and other simple practical measures. Fortunately, it is almost unknown for children to harm themselves with such activities.

Breath-holding attacks are much the most dramatic of recurrent habit patterns. Although mild attacks are quite common in children between 6 months and 5 years of age, in their most severe form, in which cerebral anoxia can cause brief generalized convulsions, they are fortunately rare. Although they are remarkably benign, it is asking a great deal of the most stoical parents to treat normally any child who carries such a devastating concealed weapon. (Breath-holding attacks are discussed in chapter 8).

Stealing

Stealing is the commonest form of delinquent behaviour, occurring in about 5 per cent of primary school children. It is a problem that particularly worries parents and teachers because of the fear that the child may later become a criminal. If, as is often the case, the stealing results in part from a feeling of rejection, the strong negative response it evokes is likely to aggravate the problem. A few incidents of stealing in a young child seldom indicate a poor long-term prognosis and an intense over-reaction from the parents of such children usually exposes their own confused and guilty feelings. However, stealing is often a feature of the behaviour of seriously deprived children and those with a more widespread antisocial pattern of behaviour. If it persists into adolescence it is clearly of more serious import.

School Problems

The most common problem is underachievement, real or imagined. The first requirement is an objective assessment of the child's true abilities. This may, of course, be difficult to achieve if the child has suffered chronic understimulation or is psychologically disturbed, but an experienced educational psychologist can generally achieve a reliable estimate and will detect specific learning problems, such as dyslexia. When these have been excluded it is necessary to look more closely at the school and the home environment to discover whether there are any problems adversely affecting the child's performance.

School refusal requires prompt firm action. It is generally a neurotic response in children and parents who are mutually anxious about separation. Such children seldom have serious social or academic problems at school. The problem is obviously self-perpetuating, and as time from school is missed it becomes progressively more difficult for the child to return. Once the general situation has been explored and any obvious environmental manipulations made, it is reasonable simply to insist that the child returns to school, to reassure his parents that he will come to no harm and to reward him strongly if he succeeds. If such simple shock tactics with positive reinforcement fail, a more comprehensive approach with the help of a psychiatrist may be required.

School truants, unlike school refusers, tend to be from homes where there is inadequate care and concern for the children, so an approach on a wide social front is likely to be necessary.

Management

When setting out to sail the poorly charted therapeutic seas of the management of behaviour problems, it is obviously important to be at least as rigorous as in approaching the better known waters of organic disease. Every doctor will evolve a personal method which should contain necessary elements within a flexible but reasonably logical framework. Although its use will become second nature, it is worthwhile stopping from time to time to examine and refurbish this structure. We will outline the steps we wish we used when approaching each new problem!

History

Since there is neither a 'right' nor 'wrong' diagnosis, nor any of the physical clues so beloved of our medical teachers, there is no possibility, as there is with organic disease, of reaching the right conclusion by a short-cut or even a totally incorrect route. The history therefore assumes special importance. It must not concentrate simply on the behaviour disturbance itself but on the antecedent factors which seem relevant when the child is considered as one element in a family and social setting. No therapeutic approach will carry weight unless the parents are convinced that the doctor has the true measure of the problem and its causes. The extraordinary success of the most popular and influential book ever written on children, Benjamin Spock's *Baby and Child Care,* has probably been due to its accurate description of all the common problems of childhood. A mother turning to its pages is soon convinced that her child's problem is not, as she feared, unique, but was only too familiar to Dr Spock. She is then well prepared to accept his advice and reassurance.

One of the most important consequences of the increasing emphasis on the child as a member of a family rather than as an isolated individual has been recognition of the fact that both parents should, whenever possible, be involved in any consideration of behaviour problems in children. Most erstwhile child psychiatrists now rightly see their role as that of family therapists and even for the amateur it is often remarkably easy, when the family is seen together, to appreciate and to help alter some of the interactions between family members which are relevant to the behaviour problems of the children.

Exclusion of Organic Disease

This vital step must not only be taken but be seen to be taken. Obviously this is particularly important when psychogenic disturbance presents in the guise of organic disease, but whenever the history reveals the least clue full physical examination and investigation are necessary. It is important to remember that, for example, general irritability and misery can be caused by coeliac disease or anaemia, sleeplessness by undetected thyrotoxicosis or asthma, temper tantrums by temporal lobe epilepsy, bowel problems by Hirschsprung's disease; the possibilities are endless and continuous vigilance is necessary. Moreover, the therapeutic powers of physical examination and simple and relatively non-invasive investigations, such as urinalysis, blood count and x-rays, should not be under-rated.

Discussion

When he has a clear picture of the problem, as much information about its cause as he can gather and is confident that there is no organic element, the general practitioner is ready to sum up and pronounce his verdict. More often than not this is the simple conclusion that the child is showing a minor and common behaviour disturbance which, in the absence of any aggravating factors, will resolve spontaneously sooner rather than later.

Treatment

If the problem is more serious further steps must be planned. These may include:

1. Family interviews for family therapy. As emphasized, these can be extraordinarily helpful and seem able to break long established maladaptive patterns remarkably quickly. The general practitioner or paediatrician will soon realize if he is out of his depth, and he can then enlist the help of a more experienced therapist.

2. Simple behaviour therapy. The art and science of obtaining desired behaviour from children through reward and punishment is practised in all households, but suitable techniques have been subjected to careful evaluation by child psychiatrists. One of the simplest devices is the widely used star chart for such problems as enuresis and encopresis. With suitable exhortation and rewards earned by accumulating stars this may be extremely effective. The principle of rewarding desired behaviour can be extended as necessary. It is sometimes helpful to plan improvements by small and easy steps. For instance, the child with an irrational fear of water may be persuaded successively to watch his friends swimming, don a swimming costume, dip a toe, paddle in the shallow end, and so on. A useful device for older children, as for adults, is the contract. This is an undertaking by the child to amend his ways, worked out by the child and the doctor by mutual agreement, then written down and signed. Children often appreciate this pleasingly elaborate and formalized game and co-operate with great enthusiasm.

3. Environmental manipulation. Clearly there are innumerable ways in which changes in the environment may help children showing behaviour disturbance. These range from simple rearrangement of a sleepless toddler's bedroom through changes of class or teacher at school to major decisions, made only after all possible avenues have been explored, such as the removal of a child from his family. Such measures are, however, adjunctive to the other aspects of management.

4. Drug treatment. Drugs have little place in the management of childhood behaviour problems. The simple placebo should not be forgotten, since at least as many children as adults are placebo responders and effective use may be made of a short course of impressive-looking inactive medication.

In sleep disorders the use of hypnotics should be limited to a few nights treatment in conjunction with other measures to break an entrenched behaviour pattern. Trichoral and Vallergan syrup are safe and effective. (For use of antidepressants in enuresis and purgatives in bowel disturbances see chapters 10 and 11.)

Affective disorders in children have not been discussed, but clearly mood disturbance will often underly disturbance of behaviour. Pathological anxiety or depression in a child requires full evaluation before drug treatment is considered.

5. More extreme sanctions. Occasionally, behaviour disturbance may require more drastic measures. The therapeutic use of admission to hospital is sometimes under-rated; a children's ward is often considered by parents less threatening than a child psychiatric unit. Very rarely, a taste of the cumbrous creaking action of the Law, in its relatively humane and flexible form of the Juvenile Courts, may be needed to urge an erring teenager back to the paths of relative righteousness! The occasional need to remove a child from home has already been mentioned.

Conclusions

The treatment of behaviour problems in children is therapeutically rewarding and, when tempted to think that an undue amount of time and trouble should not be expended on minor and self-limiting problems, it is well to reflect that there can be few more useful aspects of preventive medicine than helping to establish happy and loving relationships between parents and their children.

References and Further Reading

Bax, M. C. O., *Br. Med. J.*, 1980, **280**, 1177.

Illingworth, R. S., *The Normal Child, Some Problems of the Early Years and their Treatment,* Churchill Livingstone, Edinburgh, 1975.

Rutter, M. and Hersov, L., *Child Psychiatry, Modern Approaches,* Blackwell, Oxford, 1977.

Winnicott, D. W., *The Child and the Outside World,* Tavistock Publications, London, 1957.

17. Child Abuse

In recent years the most distressing fact which has been forced to the attention of those concerned with the care of children has been the frequency and severity with which they are maltreated by their parents and guardians. Once considered a rare aberration indeed, child abuse is now known to be an endemic disease of society, relatively unaffected by affluence and humane legislation. In historical perspective it is apparent how, over the last century, the improving public lot of children diverted attention from the failure of their private lot to improve equally. It is often pointed out that the RSPCA was founded in 1823 but the NSPCC in 1889!

The curtain of ignorance which concealed this dark corner was finally lifted in the United States in the early 1960s by Henry Kempe and his colleagues, who brought the facts to a wide general as well as medical public, not least by coining the memorable term 'battered babies'. The carnage revealed was appalling and it seemed incredible that the problem could be as great in this country. Once our eyes were opened, however, it became apparent that physical injury, soon unmemorably renamed 'non-accidental injury', was indeed common and only one aspect of the wider problem of child abuse. It is a chastening experience to read a textbook of paediatrics published more than 15 years ago. Many of the injuries and other findings now known to be typical of inflicted injury or neglect were clearly described and either accounted for in other ways or considered totally mysterious. There can be no better illustration of the axiom that, especially if the facts are unacceptable, we see only what we look for and find only what we seek.

Child abuse is a topic with wide ramifications into many areas outside medicine. In this brief account we will concentrate largely on those medical aspects which are likely to involve the family doctor.

Forms of Child Abuse

Child abuse may take many forms. The more important of these are listed in Table 17.1. Neglect is far more common than injury but the two often occur together; many, but by no means all children who are actively maltreated also suffer passive neglect. Sexual abuse of children has recently been recognized with increasing frequency and indeed, like physical injury, once sought proves surprisingly common (Tilelli et al. 1980). More subtle forms of injury caused by poisoning or inappropriate drug administration have also been described. The passive side of this coin, failure to accept or give necessary treatment, can also on occasion threaten a child's life or health. Yet another twist was provided when it was realized that some parents invent symptoms for their children and so subject them to unnecessary investigations and treatment, an aberration which has been called, clumsily, the 'Munchausen syndrome by proxy' or, obscurely, the 'Polle syndrome' (Polle was the daughter of Baron Munchausen!). Finally, interest has recently focussed on nutritional deprivation in children whose parents impose upon them strict vegetarian or other diets.

Table 17.1. Forms of child abuse.

Physical neglect, lack of food, warmth or shelter
Emotional deprivation, lack of stimulation
Physical injury, non-accidental
Sexual abuse
Poisoning or inappropriate drug administration
Withholding treatment
Munchausen syndrome by proxy, or Polle syndrome
Nutritional deprivation from rigid dietary fads

The medical approach to child abuse is beset with extremely difficult conceptual and practical problems. It has long been accepted that, within wide limits, parents should be free to treat their children as they wish; all children must be subjected to discipline and restraint; none can be given a perfect physical, intellectual and emotional environment. It is clearly impossible to define a precise point at which permissible chastisement, rough handling or sexual fondling becomes abuse or to specify exactly when poor social, nutritional or material conditions, inadequate intellectual stimulation, lack of emotional warmth or eccentric attitudes to therapy amount to frank maltreatment. Different standards are expected of families with different backgrounds and, indeed, the mores of communities change continuously. One of the results of the increasing recognition of child abuse has been that more stringent standards of child care in the home are expected and required of parents. These changes are belatedly reflected by legislation and the decisions of the courts, but the decision to intervene between a child and his parents is an extremely serious matter which has endless potential repercussions for all members of the family. It is simple only when the child's life or health is in real danger, but intervention on less tangible grounds is sometimes vital for the child's development. The social services and the courts are primarily responsible for these difficult decisions.

Incidence

The difficulties of definition and the covert nature of child abuse preclude accurate assessment of the incidence even in its most straightforward form of physical injury. Recognized abuse must represent only the tip of the iceberg but the more severe instances are likely to be those that come to light. Infants are especially at risk; two-thirds of the cases of physical injury involve those under three years of age. In England and Wales recent estimates suggest that about 100 children are killed each year and 1,500 are seriously and 5,000 moderately injured. Far more, perhaps as many as 40,000, suffer serious neglect. All social classes are represented.

In the great majority of cases it is a parent who is the aggressor and the passive partner is almost always in collusion. Adoptive and foster parents are over-represented. A small minority of children are abused by others, including cohabitees of single parents, lodgers, child minders and even occasionally siblings.

Diagnosis

Knowledge of the frequency of child abuse has, inevitably, introduced a new and unhappy element of suspicion into the approach of those concerned with children. The possibility of maltreatment must be considered when dealing with any injury, or indeed any symptom in a child for which there is not full and adequate explanation. The initial suspicion will frequently be raised not by a doctor but by a relative, neighbour, teacher, health visitor, district nurse, social worker or NSPCC representative. Once suspicion has been aroused it must be confirmed or dismissed as promptly and tactfully as possible. The general practitioner is uniquely well placed to play a central role in the assessment of this family problem because of his knowledge of the whole family and the ease with which he can enter the home and examine the children. On the other hand few general practitioners will have much personal experience of child abuse since, on average, they can expect to come across only one serious case every four or five years.

The warning signs are sometimes subtle indeed but more frequently they are obvious and stereotyped. Clinical clues to the problem encompass a very wide range but we have tried to set out some of the more important ones in Table 17.2 under the headings of the social background, the history and the child. We will now consider these in a little more detail.

The Social Background

The multiple problems of the cycle of deprivation are all too frequently a legacy from one generation to another. Many parents involved in child abuse have themselves come from deprived and violent backgrounds. They are often very young, of limited intelligence and totally inexperienced in parenthood, and yet have to cope in circumstances and on an income that would tax the best manager. Additional stresses imposed by marital discord, unwanted pregnancy, illness or unemployment can easily overwhelm their personal and material resources. It is surprising how many such couples manage to remain buoyant in spite of all their problems and how few sink into debt, despair and violence. It is important also to remember that child abuse can and does occur in affluent households.

The History

The history of a child's injuries or symptoms may strongly suggest the possibility of abuse. The most obvious and most common clue is failure of the story offered to explain the observed injuries. Children seldom sustain multiple injuries in household falls. (However, some children are remarkably accident-prone and accidents are the most frequent cause of death in the one to 14 year age-group.) Inconsistency of the history on retelling, or between members of the family, must also raise suspicion. Even when a semi-plausible account is given by one member, the anger, guilt and confusion surrounding the events has generally precluded careful rehearsal of an alibi and to expose inaccuracies and inconsistencies does not require the skills of a leading prosecuting counsel. More subtle historical clues include 'cries for help', such as multiple consultations for trivial problems concerning the child and expressed dislike and fear of damaging him. Some help in voicing these feelings may be needed; questions such as 'do you really feel fond of this child?' or 'do you

Table 17.2. Clinical clues to child abuse.

1. The social background

Parental problems including:
- Youth and immaturity
- Single parent, forced marriage, marital breakdown or violence
- Low intelligence, inadequacy, drug or alcohol dependence
- Deprived or violent upbringing
- Unemployment or illness
- Frequent pregnancies, exhaustion, depression
- Aggressive or criminal tendencies

Environmental problems including:
- Overcrowding, poor housing
- Poverty, debt
- Isolation

2. The history

Inadequate or inconsistent explanation of lesions or symptoms

Delay in presentation

Multiple consultation for minor symptoms

Expressed fear of damaging child or inability to cope

Derogatory comments concerning the child, 'scapegoat' in sibship

Pre-, peri- and postnatal problems including:
- Unwanted pregnancy
- Neglect of antenatal care
- Difficult delivery
- Preterm of small-for-dates baby
- Neonatal illness
- Mother/baby separation

Reluctance to permit examination

3. The child

Unkempt child

Behaviour disturbance including:
- Unresponsiveness
- Frozen watchfulness, fear of adults
- 'Naughtiness', hyperactivity
- Prolonged screaming

Unexplained problems, such as:
- Failure to gain weight or grow
- Developmental retardation
- Symptoms in any system

Physical injury including:
- Multiple or repeated injuries
- Bruises, cuts, abrasions, oral injury
- Burns, scalds
- Intraocular, intracranial bleeding
- Genital, anal injuries
- Fractures

ever fear you may lose control and injure him?' may open a floodgate of distress. Sometimes it becomes apparent that one sibling has been given, or has taken on the role of scapegoat for all his siblings' misdemeanours. Another surprisingly common feeling among parents who abuse their children is the conviction that the child's behaviour was calculated to distress them; 'he does it just to annoy me' is a statement frequently made about a crying infant. Similarly the parents may reveal totally unrealistic expectations for the child's age over, for instance, table manners or toilet training.

Pre-, peri- and postnatal problems are common in abused children and a history of difficulties, especially prolonged separation of mother and baby and failure of 'bonding', during these sensitive periods is ominous.

The Child

The general state of the child may, but often does not, indicate that he is inadequately cared for (Figure 17.1). His behaviour may be withdrawn and obviously fearful of adults or it may be misleadingly normal. The state of 'frozen watchfulness' sometimes adopted by children who have been physically maltreated is characteristic and can be very striking (Figure 17.2).

Infants who scream incessantly are sometimes battered and indeed it may be difficult to determine whether the behaviour is the result or the cause of the maltreatment. Similarly, badly behaved older children invite more than usually firm restraint, which can escalate into violence. Much that has been written on child abuse fails to acknowledge the fact that the transaction is not entirely one-sided. Some infants and children, if not exactly inviting maltreatment, are very much more aggravating than others and their behaviour cannot be ascribed entirely to parental attitudes. The mildest parent of the happiest child is occasionally provoked to intense anger and clearly the combination of an unusually difficult child with a volatile and potentially violent parent may be explosive. Parents who are feeling guilty and distressed may appreciate being reminded of these obvious facts.

Deprived children often show retarded growth and development without evidence of underlying organic disease. Many factors, including inadequate intake, secondary endocrine disturbance and lack of stimulation, are involved (see chapter 1). Growth in height and, to a greater extent, weight are affected. Proof of the diagnosis requires removal of the child to a more suitable environment in which remarkable 'catch-up' growth may occur. Psychomotor progress may also show global retardation with speech and social functions generally more retarded than motor skills. The extent to which a child catches up can be equally remarkable once appropriate stimulation is given.

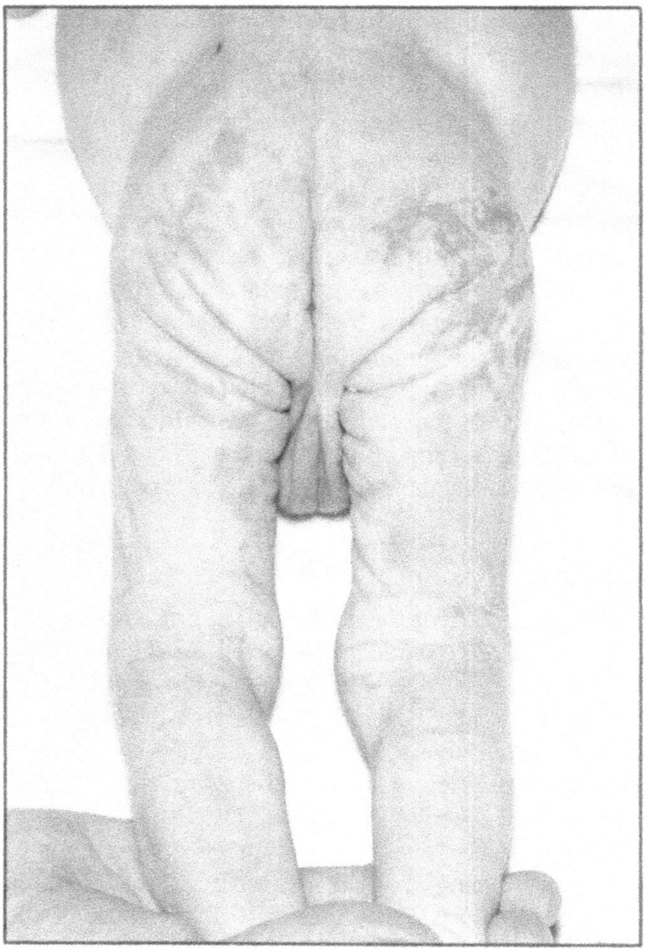

Figure 17.1. *The tail end (often the most revealing aspect) of a malnourished neglected child.*

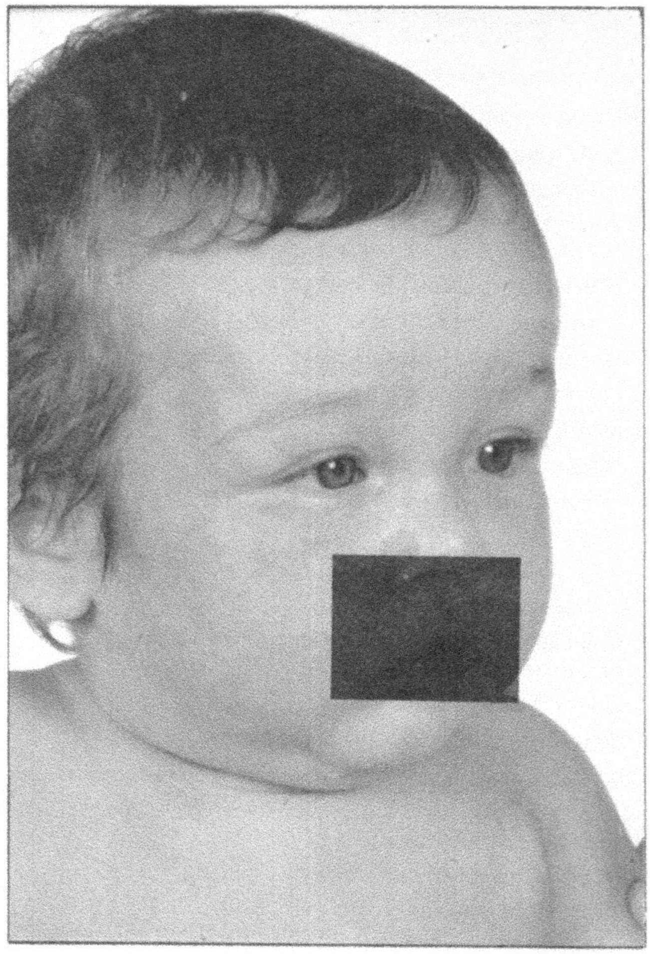

Figure 17.2. *An abused child showing facial bruising and 'frozen watchfulness'.*

When a child presents with obscure symptoms for which full investigation fails to reveal a cause, the possibility of maltreatment should be considered. We have encountered children with hypernatraemia (fatal in one case) from administration of salt, coma from barbiturates, fainting from diuretics, and recurrent conjunctivitis from the instillation of irritants. We have also investigated children for fits, haematemesis and haemoptysis which proved to be factitious.

However, much the most frequent indicator of non-accidental injury is the occurrence of bruising and other skin lesions due to violent handling. If these occur repeatedly it is, of course, especially worrying but it is important to remember that children can be as severely injured by parents who only occasionally lose control as by those who are habitually violent. Accidentally acquired injuries are rare in infancy but almost universal in children learning to walk. These tend, however, to be confined to certain areas such as the forehead, knees and shins. Lesions especially suspicious of non-accidental injury include the following.

Finger Tip Bruises

These are caused by gripping the child with excessive force and are most often seen on the trunk, the proximal parts of the limbs (Figure 17.3) and around the mouth (Figure 17.4). There may be a row of up to four small round bruises sometimes with an opposing thumb bruise. Deliberate pinch marks are similar.

Other Bruises and Abrasions

The form of the lesions may suggest beating with straps, cords (Figure 17.5) or other flexible objects or contact with hard surfaces, such as walls or pieces of furniture. A black eye is an unusual accidental lesion because the orbit protects the eye from contact with a flat surface and two black eyes, in the absence of massive bruising of the forehead, are especially suspicious (Figure 17.6). A tear of the upper or lower lip frenulum or abrasion within the mouth is a characteristic injury which can be missed. Lesions of the genitalia and perianal region are infrequently accidentally acquired and must be viewed with suspicion (Figure 17.7).

Bites

Bites characteristically cause bruising, with or without puncturing the skin, in two semicircular rows separated by about an inch (Figure 17.8). Siblings on the offensive (or defensive) often consider the teeth a fair weapon, presumably because they were provided by nature, so the size of the indentation must be taken into account!

Burns and Scalds

The small, often multiple, circular burns caused by cigarettes are typical lesions of non-accidental injury. Burns resulting from pressure against heating elements are also characteristic. Scalding is common and often affects the distal parts of limbs in glove or stocking distribution when they have been forced into hot water (Figure 17.9). It may also affect the buttocks and perineum when, usually during battles over toilet training, the child has been forced to sit in hot water.

Figure 17.3. *Circumferential bruising of a limb from violent handling.*

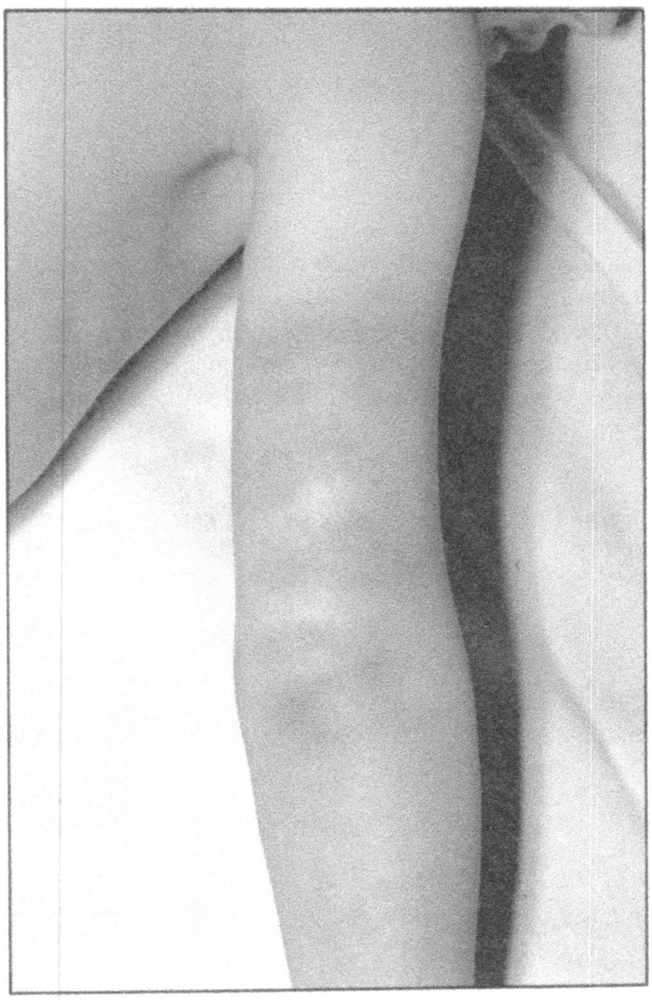

Head Injuries

Head injuries may result in intracranial bleeding with or without skull fracture. Retinal haemorrhage is a characteristic physical sign. It may result from violent shaking (Figure 17.10) as well as from direct injury.

Fractures

Fractures are common and often occur in characteristic patterns. Multiple bony injuries at different stages of healing are very suspicious. Multiple rib fractures, skull fractures, injuries to the metaphyses of long bones, displacement of the epiphyses and subperiosteal bleeding are among the most typical skeletal injuries.

Management

Considering the problem of potential and actual child abuse in broad context, every general practitioner must be aware of many families about which he feels concern. To judge the appropriate action in each case obviously requires assessment of many factors but, for the purpose of discussion, we will consider three levels of anxiety.

Mild Anxiety

Into this category are likely to fall a large number of families with major social and psychological problems in which there has been no direct evidence of child abuse in any form. As much practical and emotional support as possible needs to be mobilized. The general practitioner is unlikely to be able to devote a great deal of his time to this and his health visitor is probably the first person on whom he will call. The enlistment of further support from a social worker will often be necessary. For the young, impoverished and isolated mother of preschool children often the most useful measure is to arrange for the children to attend a local authority play group or nursery so that mother and children are permitted regular respite from each other's company. Many other practical measures may be helpful. Regular contact with the family by a member of the primary health care team will not only provide help and support but will also allow the doctor to receive prompt notice if the children show signs of abuse or the general situation deteriorates.

Moderate Anxiety

This emotion is likely to arise in the breast of the conscientious general practitioner when he suspects that

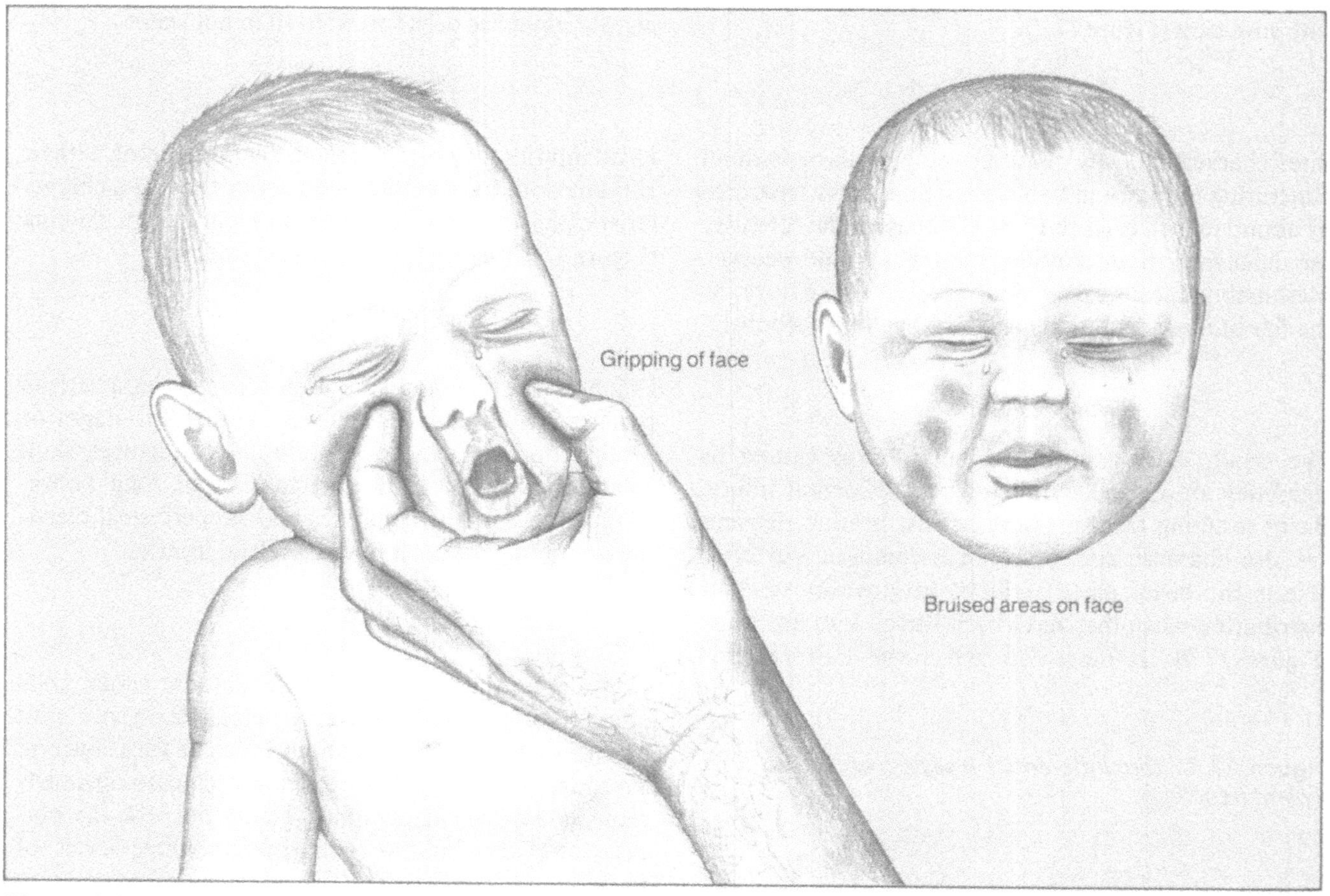

Figure 17.4. *Rough attempts to quieten a crying child often leave finger tip bruises around the mouth.*

a child is suffering maltreatment but has little direct evidence. The family clearly needs the regular attention of a health visitor and a social worker. Other agencies which may usefully be involved include the NSPCC and the community medicine services. It may also prove useful to have the child assessed by a paediatrician. Fortunately few parents object to a 'specialist opinion' on their child's growth and development and admission to hospital for 'investigation', often in fact simply for observation, is also generally acceptable.

The cornerstone of the management of child abuse problems, however, is the much derided but invaluable case discussion or, in its formal guise, the case conference. This event ensures that all the people involved with helping and supporting a family come together to present the aspects known to them. Almost invariably a far clearer picture of the problem emerges and a sensible plan can be formulated. One of the most important features of such a plan is the appointment of one worker as the primary agent or key worker responsible for the family. A 'lifeline' to a reliable and supportive person, who visits regularly and can be called upon whenever the parents reach the stage of desperation in which they fear they may harm the child, is invaluable and may be life-saving.

Many doctors, used to making their own rather than participating in committee decisions, at first find working as a member of a 'multidisciplinary team' highly

Figure 17.5. *Lesions caused by beating with a double cord.*

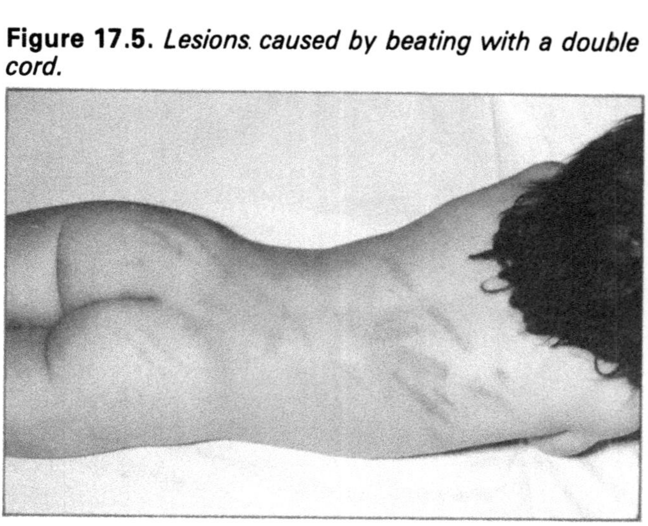

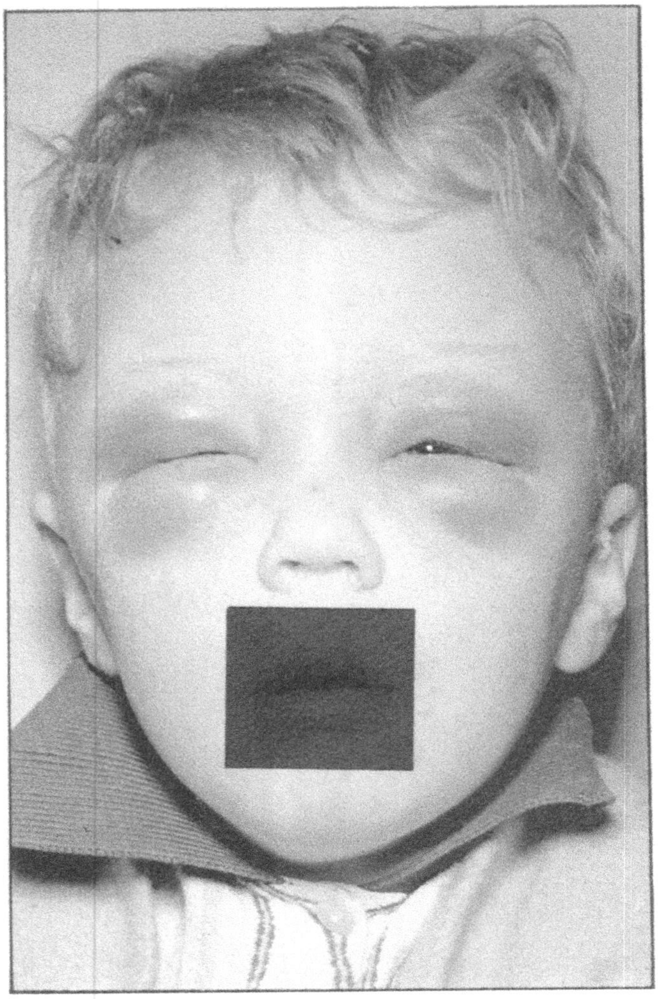

Figure 17.6. *Two black eyes, a very suspicious pattern of injury in a child.*

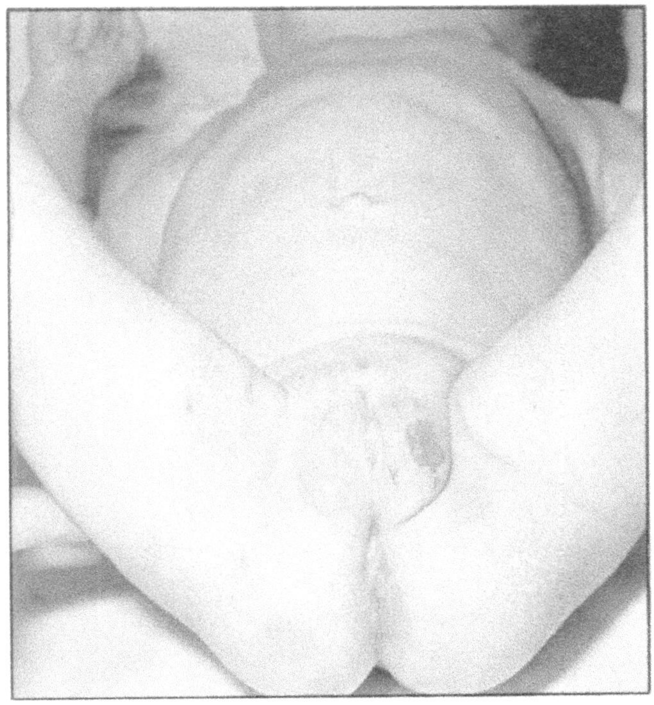

Figure 17.7. *Perineal lesions resulting from sexual abuse in an infant.*

irksome and we have all, at some time, calculated the cost of a case conference in terms of the summed salaries of those present! However, the decisions involved in cases of child abuse require the fullest possible assessment of the problem and are far too difficult, and indeed legally compromising, for any one person to make. A case conference should, at the least, provide a fuller understanding of the problem and clear directives on how and by whom the family is to be helped and supervised.

Severe Anxiety

What action is appropriate if there is evidence, or strong suspicion, that a child is suffering maltreatment and is really in danger? The child must first be removed from the home environment. Admission to hospital is nearly always the simplest and most acceptable way for this end to be achieved although there are alternatives, such as removal to relatives or admission to a local authority children's home. If the parents refuse to permit such action a Place of Safety Order must be obtained. This requires the signature of a magistrate and permits removal of the child to a place of safety for up to 28 days. All social service departments are familiar with the procedure for obtaining such orders.

On the child's admission to hospital routine measures include careful examination for signs of neglect or injury and photographic recording of any present, a skeletal survey to detect evidence of old or new bony injury, and appropriate investigations to exclude a bruising or bleeding tendency or any other underlying organic problem. An early case conference must be called and representatives of all agencies must attend. The decision of the case conference is likely to include adding the child's name to the child abuse register which is maintained in all health districts (and to which general practitioners have access) and it may be decided that legal proceedings must be taken against the parents. Application to the Juvenile Court either for a Supervision or a Care Order is then made. There are several variations on these themes, ranging from voluntary supervision of the family without statutory right of access to the home to compulsory admission into care with the local authority taking over all parental rights. Discussion of the legal niceties is outside the scope of this chapter but doctors involved with these distressing cases should have some idea of the working of the

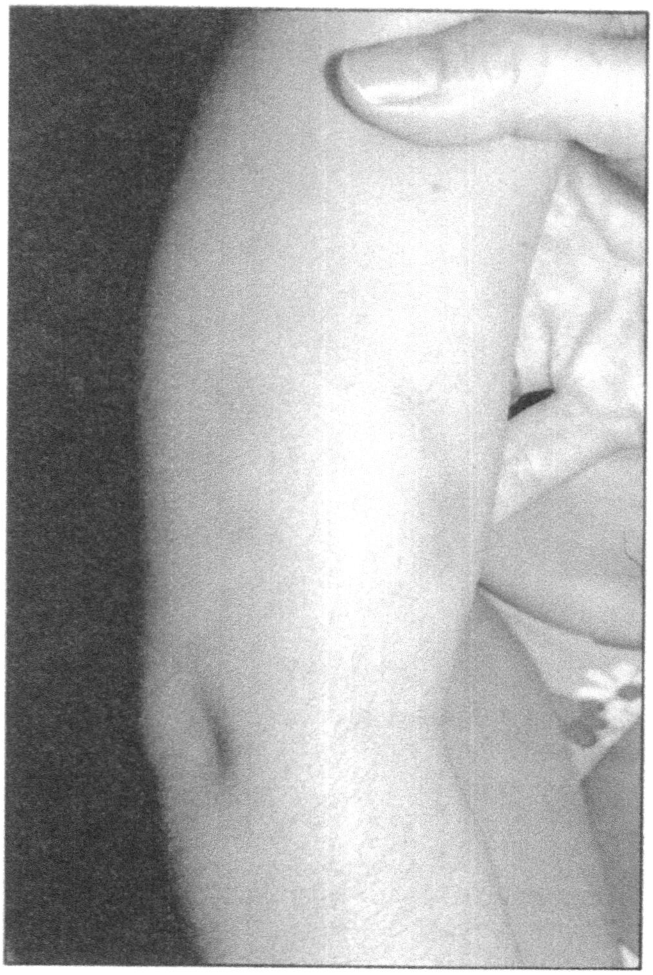

Figure 17.8. *A typical bite mark.*

Juvenile Court, in which various modifications of the normal rules of evidence apply. A good short but comprehensive and, to legal laymen, comprehensible account can be found in Hall and Mitchell (1978).

Figure 17.9. *The scalded and bruised hand of an injured child.*

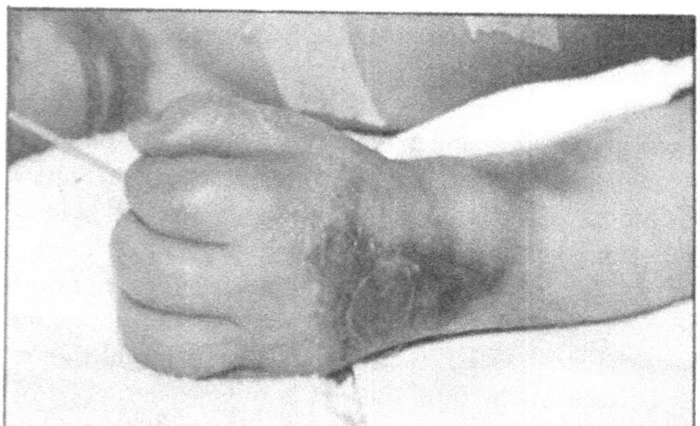

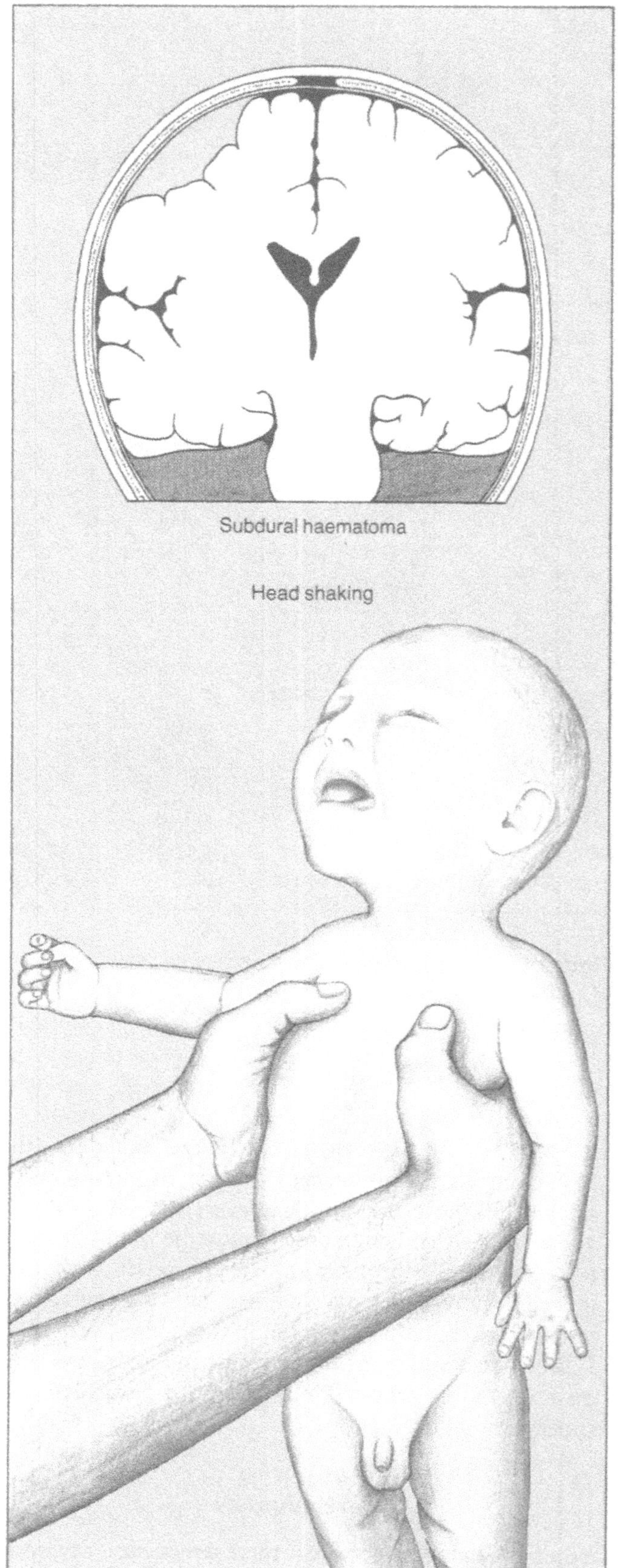

Figure 17.10. *Violent shaking may cause intracranial and retinal bleeding.*

Prevention

Recent interest and concern over the problem of child abuse has led to fuller understanding of the many factors which combine to place a child at risk of maltreatment. It is often possible, at a case conference on a battered child, to build up a picture of the roots of the problem extending back through the childhood of the parents to previous generations, and to see clearly how accumulated frustration and despair culminated in the circumstances in which a crying child was wounded or killed. Increasing experience of these problems seems to us to emphasize more and more that the parents are victims not villains. A similar change in attitude from incomprehension and horror to understanding and sympathy has been apparent not only among the social services and other caring professions but also among the police.

Since the roots of the problem are embedded in the structure of society a broad approach to prevention must encompass a wide social and political attack on the cycle of deprivation and on the many ways our present society fails to support, educate and maintain the physical and mental health of its members in their reproductive and childrearing role. Development of this large thesis does not fall within the modest confines of this chapter. There are, however, practical measures that can be taken by the general practitioner in this area. Perhaps most important is the promotion of good antenatal instruction and perinatal care. Recent research has re-emphasized the enormous importance of early 'bonding' in the mother-child relationship and the poor prognosis if this attachment process fails. For many mothers attachment is far from instant and they should be warned that this is often the case. Close supervision and support should be provided if, for any reason, the process fails. Through his ancillary helpers, especially the health visitors, the general practitioner can have considerable influence on preparation for and instruction in parenthood. He can also do his best to see that all appropriate welfare services are made available to those in need.

On a more immediate level hope of prevention lies in identification of families in need and anticipation of their problems before a crisis is reached. The major pointers to danger were summarized in Table 17.2. The most important single measure is probably, as emphasized above, the provision of a reliable person on whom the parents can call when in need of help. This does not necessarily have to be a professionally trained and salaried member of the social or health services and imaginative solutions, such as the use of 'surrogate grannies' have been tried with apparent success in the USA. Of almost equal importance is to ensure that parent and child have some time free from each other's company. This can be achieved by the use of child minders, baby sitters, playgroups, day care and nurseries but, once again, more informal arrangements may work equally well.

Mother and child should also be encouraged to get out of the house together. This can sometimes be combined with education in baby and child care through regular visits to the clinic, mother and toddler groups and, where available, classes in mothercraft. Help with practical matters, such as obtaining housing and all the financial assistance to which the welfare state entitles them, is obviously important. A home help may be needed and can be used as an educational and emotionally supportive as well as a purely practical helper.

The parents may require treatment of their own health problems, advice on contraception, marriage guidance or psychiatric treatment. Unfortunately, provision of help along these lines may prove difficult and somewhat thankless work. In many areas there is a severe shortage of facilities for children. The stretched social, medical and psychiatric services tend to have little time for preventive work and, almost by definition, many families at risk are resistant even to the most tactful and thoughtful attempts to give assistance.

Much criticism, only in part constructive, has been directed at the professionals who were considered to have failed in their preventive role by one of the many enquiries which have been set up to investigate the more spectacular cases of child abuse to reach the public eye. It is perhaps well to remember, finally, that diversion of infinite funds and personnel to this problem would fail to eradicate it. The best safeguard for children is informed awareness of the problem, good communication and prompt action when necessary but, inevitably, some failures will occur.

Reference

Hall, J. G. and Mitchell, B. A., *Child Abuse—Procedure and Evidence in Juvenile Courts,* Barry Rose Ltd, Chichester, 1978.

Tilelli, J. A., Turek, D. and Jaffe, A. C., *New Engl. J. Med.,* 1980, **302,** 319.

Further Reading

Franklin, A. W., *Child Abuse,* Churchill Livingstone, Edinburgh, 1978.

Kempe, H. S. and Kempe, C. H., *Child Abuse,* Harvard University Press, 1978.

Taylor, L. and Newberger, E. H., *New Engl. J. Med.,* 1979, **301,** 1205.

Index

GPSR Compliance
The European Union's (EU) General Product Safety Regulation (GPSR) is a set of rules that requires consumer products to be safe and our obligations to ensure this.

If you have any concerns about our products, you can contact us on

ProductSafety@springernature.com

In case Publisher is established outside the EU, the EU authorized representative is:

Springer Nature Customer Service Center GmbH
Europaplatz 3
69115 Heidelberg, Germany

www.ingramcontent.com/pod-product-compliance
Ingram Content Group UK Ltd.
Pitfield, Milton Keynes, MK11 3LW, UK
UKHW051004220926
475831UK00003B/111
9789400974265